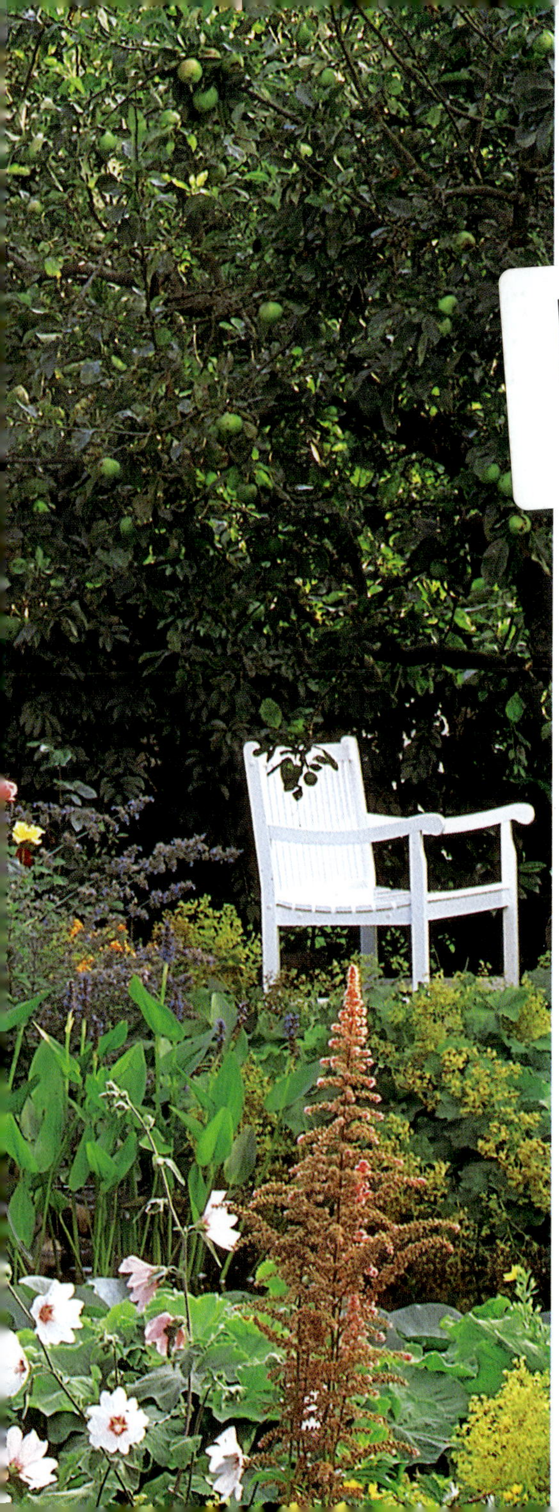

Success with Feng Shui f… arden

GÜNTHER SATOR

Editor

KAREN DOUTHWAITE

MEREHURST

Introduction

Good energy for you and your garden

The ancient Far-Eastern teachings of feng shui are beginning to capture the imagination of more and more Westerners. The aim of feng shui is to create an harmonious flow of energies that will have a positive influence on the whole of one's life. This book is about feng shui in the garden. It offers an introduction to the principles and wisdom of this ancient tradition and also gives you the information you need to design and create a feng shui garden from scratch, plus many useful tips on how to redesign an existing garden.

Using simple, practical examples, feng shui expert Günther Sator shows you how to ensure that good energy flows in your garden. There is a pull-out plan (p. 16), showing you how to find the all-important 'bagua' zones in your garden – each one relating to a different aspect of your life. Using the bagua plan alongside the easy-reference tables and questionnaires will make it easy for you to determine the energy zones and any changes that may be necessary in your garden. The book's stunning colour photographs and clear illustrations will give you many more hints and ideas about the kinds of plants and accessories you can use to strengthen individual areas of the garden and balance out its deficiencies.

Contents

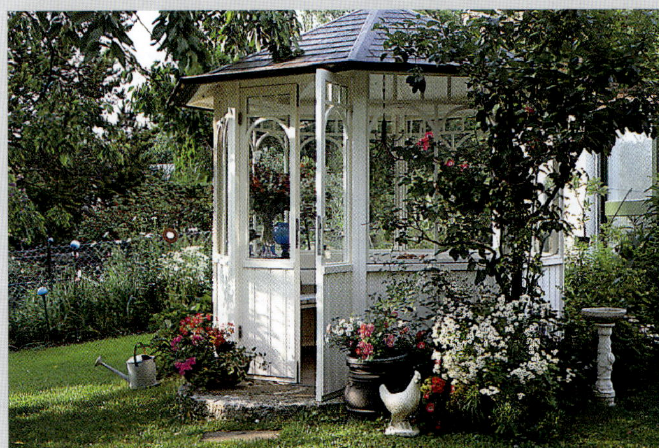

Relax in a flower-decked pavilion.

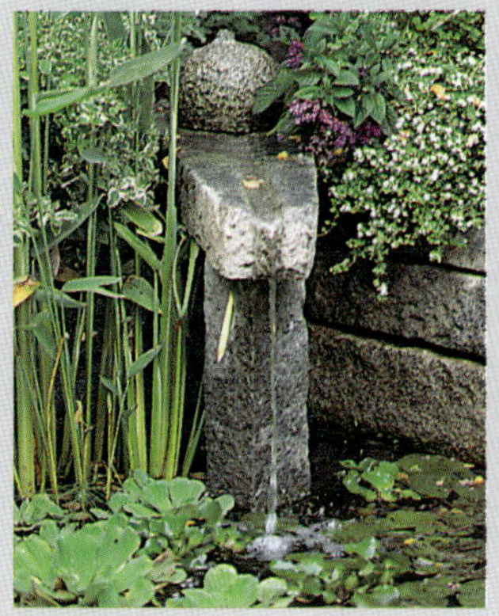

Refreshing water.

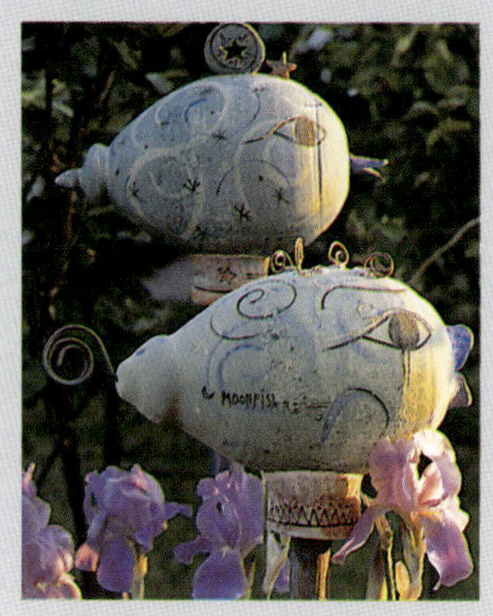

Well-chosen accessories.

The ideal feng shui garden appeals to all five senses, not just to our sense of sight, so this book explains how a few simple changes can stimulate our senses of hearing, touch, taste and smell – doing wonders for our appreciation of the garden. Wishing you much enjoyment and every success with feng shui in your garden.

The author

Günther Sator is the first European feng shui consultant to design a practical approach to the teachings of feng shui, tailoring it specifically to meet the demands of our modern Western lifestyle.

The photographers

The colour photographs are by well-known photographers (see p. 63) who have worked on numerous other books in the *Success With* series.

The illustrator

Marlene Gemke studied graphic design at the Fachhochschule Wiesbaden and then became a freelance scientific illustrator. She has contributed to many of the other titles in the *Success With* series.

Important: Please pay particular attention to the *Warning and notes* on p. 63 so you may enjoy your feng shui garden to the full and in complete safety.

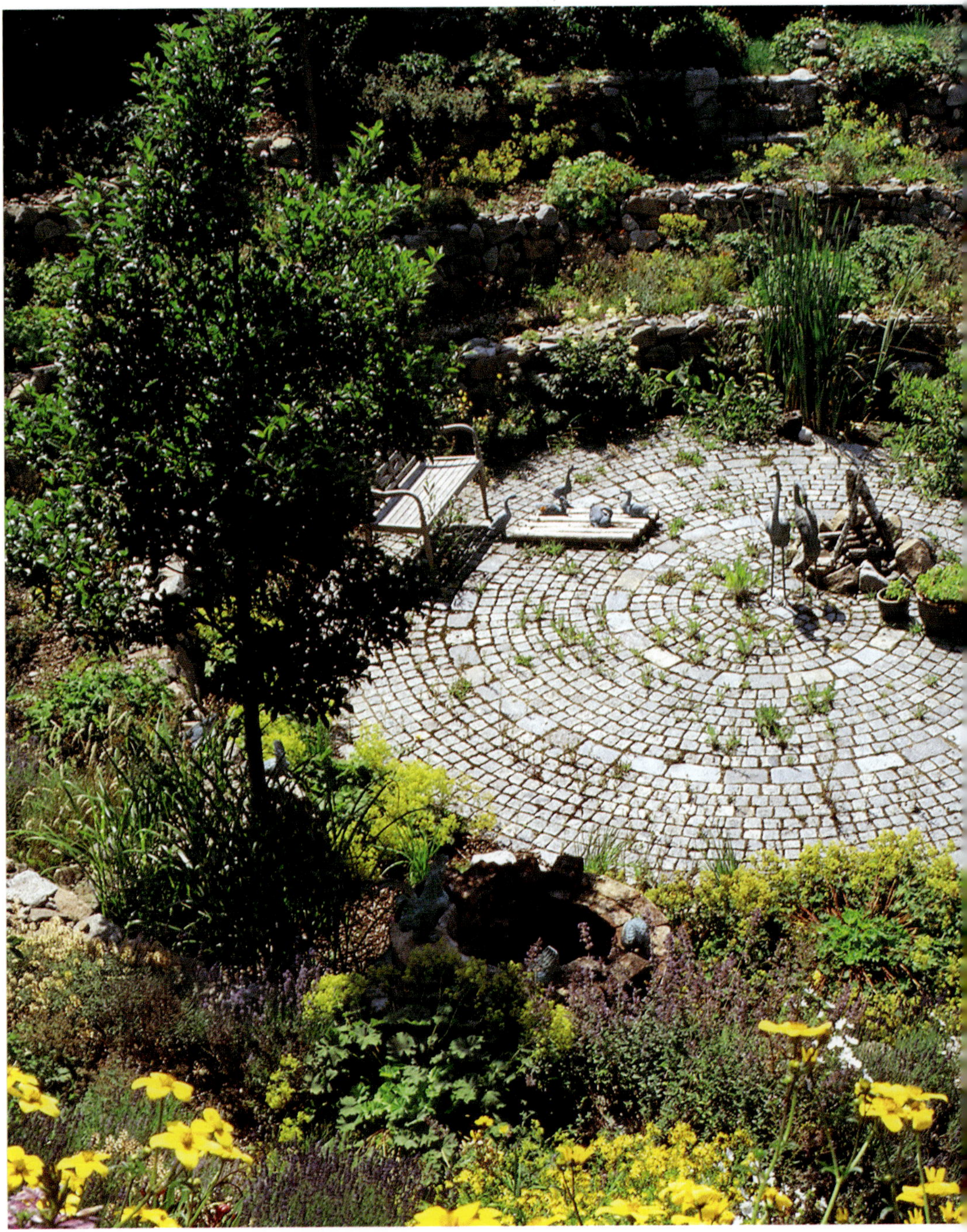

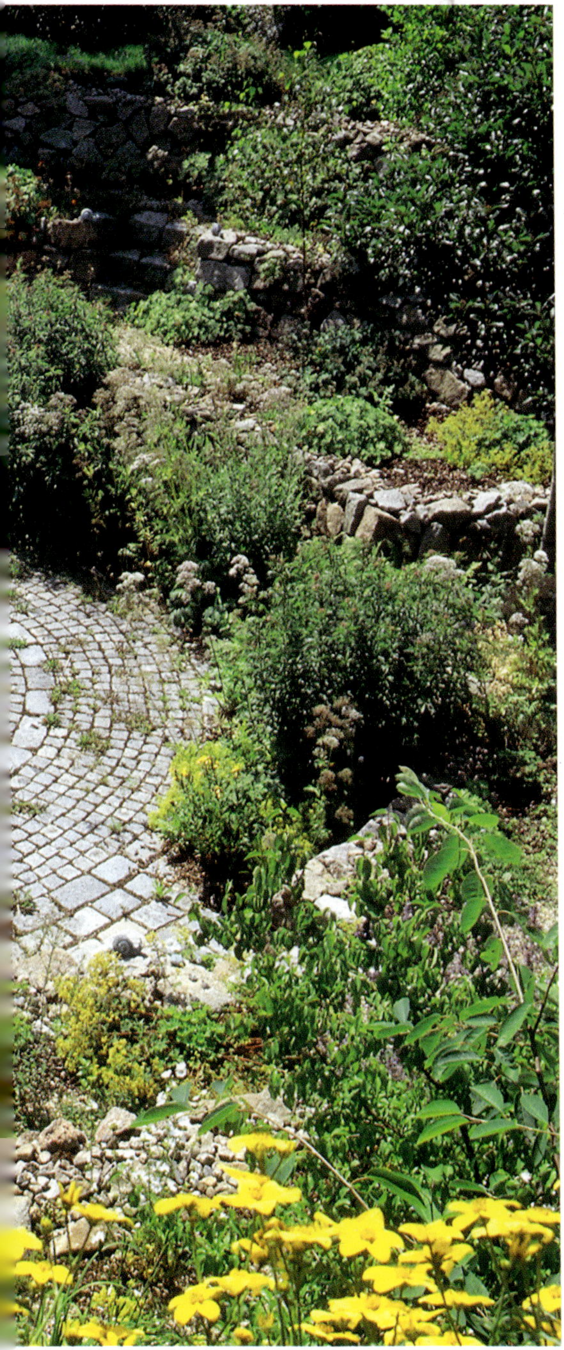

Ancient wisdom

What is Feng Shui?

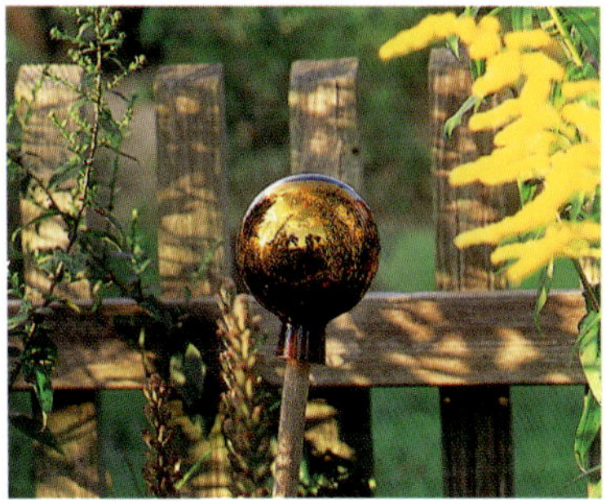

Reflecting gazing or mirror balls collect energy and inhibit harmful influences.

The Far-Eastern teaching known as feng shui (pronounced fung shway) is based on a tradition thousands of years old. It evolved from Man's close contact with nature and his attempts to explain nature's workings. In this book we look at the origins of feng shui and at how its ancient theories can be put into practice in our modern Western lifestyles.

A sunken sitting area gives a sense of security and makes small gardens look much larger.

Ancient wisdom

'Man and his environment are one' according to an old Chinese proverb. Our ancestors, too, knew that the fate of Man was closely dependent on his surroundings. The daily weather conditions affected and defined their everyday lives, while the surrounding vegetation and the shape of the landscape, with all its protective features, were of great importance.

Very gradually the knowledge that Man had gained through experience, observation and from his intuitive responses to the signs of nature was passed on to succeeding generations. This process was not just happening in the Far East, but in every region of the world.

All the ancient cultures developed similar ideas about the 'spirit of nature'. Legends that have been handed down to us concerning the beginning of the world indicate that these ideas referred to a 'greater whole' behind the visible world. The Native Americans' songs about the Great Spirit, for example, sounded very similar to the stories told around the camp fires of bushmen in Central Africa and the aborigines in Australia. They observed the world with awe and gratitude and believed it was created by and inhabited by this higher being (sometimes several beings). They tried as well as they could to live in harmony with this almighty power, as departing from the chosen path would have meant plunging into disharmony and dire misfortune. Prayers were offered to the creator of all life and our ancestors showed their humility and reverence in all everyday activities.

Different types of 'geomancy' arose from these experiences, depending on the culture concerned. Geomancy means 'earth prophecy' but it also concerns the harmonious relations between man, his buildings and structures and nature surrounding them. Feng shui is a special form of this geomancy – translated literally feng shui means 'wind and water' – which developed in particular throughout Tibet and China and its traditional teachings are still practised today. Western geomantic tradition, on the other hand, has unfortunately been lost over the centuries and this is one reason why feng shui is becoming increasingly popular and important in the West.

Feng shui for the West

It is important to find a way of converting and adapting the teachings of feng shui to suit our surroundings and culture. The classical elements of Chinese garden architecture, such as a pagoda, Asiatic plants, or a colourful dragon sculpture guarding an entrance would probably look too exotic and rather out of place in most Western gardens and, without the proper cultural references to support them, these features would not really fulfil the purposes assigned to them. That is why this book concentrates exclusively on European garden design suggestions and the background and reasons for them will be explained.

Chi – the life energy

We must all have experienced the calming effects that a sparkling stream has on us as it meanders gently through the landscape. By contrast, a murky, stagnant canal encased in concrete will appear quite cheerless. This is due to the distinctly different quality of life energy in these two types of water courses, the universal energy that gives life to everything that surrounds us. In feng shui this energy is called chi and it is of central importance to our understanding of the basic techniques. It is a similar concept to the breath of life of the Great Spirit in the belief systems of ancient cultures.

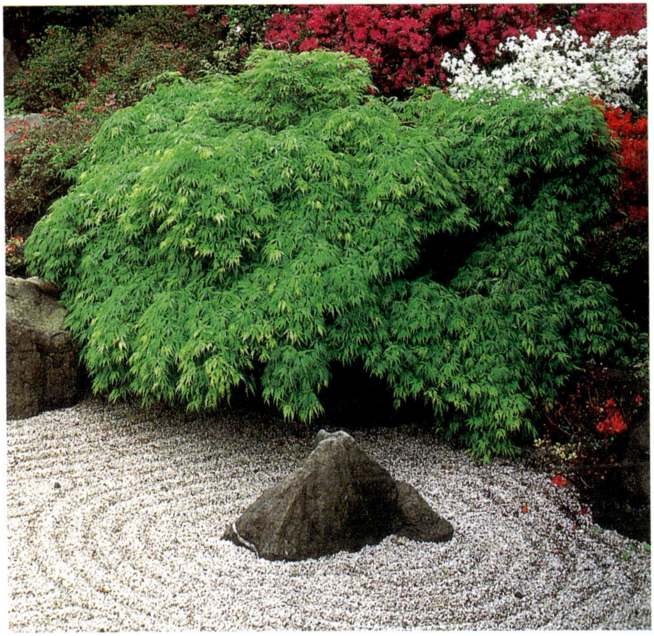

A classical Japanese garden, with raked gravel.

Chi is invisible yet omnipresent. Chi is the cause and effect of everything, no matter whether it is hidden away or directly observable. Chi is the essence that causes mountains to form, that saturates the air and which we perceive whenever we feel particularly full of well-being in a certain place. Even apparently lifeless objects like stones or garden accessories are made of this basic substance and should, therefore, be perceived as living – although, admittedly, this is a slightly unusual idea for us to grasp, with our view of the world rooted as it is in the hard facts of scientific thought.

The garden as a microcosm

The world functions according to clear-cut rules where energy is concerned, in the Western world as well as in China or Tibet. One of the basic rules of life is constant change, something that can be seen clearly in the garden as it is governed by very obvious seasonal changes. Tomorrow nothing will be exactly the same as it is today, even if it appears so superficially. Energy must move constantly, as otherwise it would come to a standstill. According to Chinese medicine, whenever a free flow of energy is prevented in our bodies this will cause weaknesses in our health. A building, too, may suffer from a deficiency in energy flow which will then be reflected in the fate of its occupants.
In a similar way, an harmonious flow of chi energy should be possible in a garden and its nourishing potential will, in turn, have a beneficial, fortifying effect on the surroundings and the people living in it. It enhances well-being and also makes it easier to lead a happy and successful life.
The ideal situation, of course, would be to use feng shui in the home and the garden so that both inside and outside there can be a positive, beneficial influence on different areas of one's life (see p. 16).

What is feng shui?

Traditional garden design

Planning gardens according to geomantic principles is a long tradition which exists all over the world. Apart from being agreeable to look at, a garden in which the basic needs of nature have been considered develops a special aura that makes it extremely easy to recuperate and find inspiration there. Harmonious green areas also have a healing effect on their surroundings and nearby buildings and will also noticeably improve the micro-climate.

Ancient knowledge in monastery gardens

Even in the West, monastery gardens as well as many traditional knot gardens and even some parks have been designed in a way that encourages an harmonious energy flow. The arrangement of flower-beds and connecting paths, the choice of the right types of plants and their combinations and also the careful placing of chi-enhancing features like gazing balls or fountains were carried out according to old and well-known principles that are still in use to this day.

Modern garden architecture

Even though this ancient knowledge still exists, modern garden architecture does not seem to value it very highly and tends to overlook completely the energy-giving powers of gardens. Hundreds of thousands of gardens and parks have been planted with the same kind of dull and unimaginative greenery. Gardens like these are designed to be low-maintenance but generally their appearance is sterile and only in very few cases do they present an harmonious total picture. The living chi withers in such surroundings and the result merely emphasises the dreariness of the existing living and working conditions.

Feng shui gardens

Even the smallest green area can serve as an extended living area and if designed properly according to the principles of feng shui, will cheer the visitor with nurturing and fortifying chi energy. You do not even need to step into this type of green paradise: just looking at it from a window in your home may enrich your life on a continuous daily basis. You will be surprised at the positive effects this may have upon your psyche and general physical well-being over the years. Even in the winter, when you look at a garden lying in a deep winter sleep, a feng shui garden will demonstrate its harmonising powers.

Important: In this book the term 'feng shui garden' refers to a Western style garden, purposely designed according to the needs of an harmonious energy flow and the rules of nature, not to a copied classical Chinese garden.

Acupuncture in the garden

The ideal feng shui garden consists of elements that are as simple as possible and will allow a free, harmonious energy flow in all directions. To achieve this the surroundings of the garden have to be incorporated in the total plan. The actual size of the garden will not play a great part as the inner structure of a feng shui garden and its link with the outside world will be unfolded according to the same rules and principles whatever the area of space. Every plant, every stone, every design element functions as an energy focus. They have a very similar function to that of acupuncture needles on the meridian lines of the human body.

Just as a total detoxification programme often forms the beginning of a course of therapy, one of the first steps undertaken in an established garden will often be to detoxify it, removing any excesses to recreate a balance and enable the chi to circulate freely. A feng shui garden should be a happy place with plenty of good chi to spare. Wherever possible, make use of the garden's existing structure and take advantage of any good features. The starting point for planning is the plot of ground and its surroundings, and the good and bad influences they present. As we will see, it is relatively easy to subdue the bad influences. Another important feature is the main entrance to the site through which a great deal of chi will enter. The building, with its connection to the garden, and the view from your windows both play important roles. You will find out more about this in the following pages.

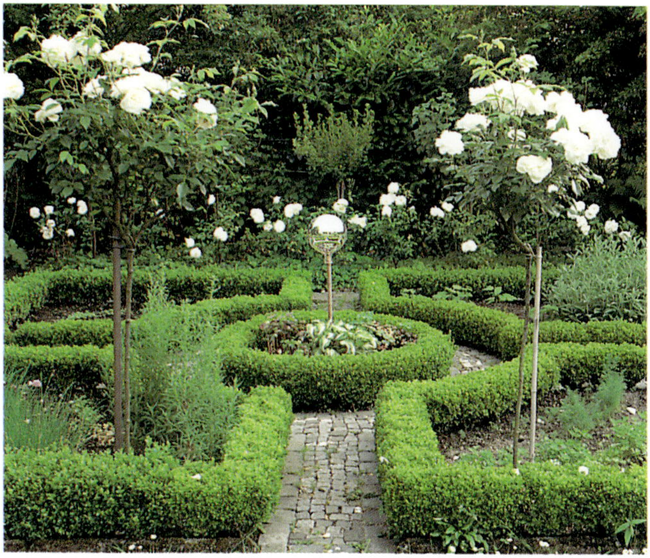

A knot garden with a reflecting gazing ball in the centre.

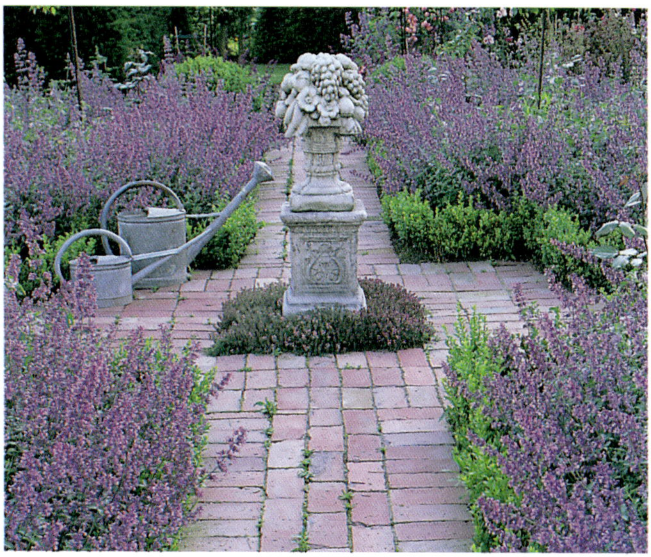

Monastery gardens typically have a strong focal point in the centre.

The ideal garden

You should see your piece of land as one complete unit – this may mean including the house itself in your feng shui scheme. If the house divides the land into two distinct gardens you may wish to treat these separately. However, as feng shui is all about balance and harmony, it is best to find a way of bringing these 'separate' areas together, to give more unity to your garden and your life.

The ideal shape for a feng shui garden is a rectangle or square, preferably on a level plot of ground. The best position is facing the sun – in our Northern Hemisphere that would be facing roughly to the south. Not all gardens will match these feng shui ideals, but the art is to work with the advantages and play down the disadvantages.

- The more irregularly shaped and rugged a plot is, the more restlessness and disturbance will appear in the lives of the people living there. This should not necessarily be viewed as negative, as people employed in creative activities will often feel a great deal more comfortable in such surroundings. You can also use some feng shui rules to create a balance (see p. 12).
- Sloping gardens, particularly steep ones, need special handling (see p. 30) so that not too much of the vital chi runs down the slope and gets lost.
- One suggestion is to lay the bagua plan (see p. 16-22) over a plan of your garden in order to find out more about its possible effects on you and your family. The bagua will provide information on which aspects of your life are either particularly weak or particularly emphasised.

Cutting chi

Even with the life energy of chi, too much of a good thing can be unhealthy. If it is allowed to run along straight roads or paths it becomes too concentrated and harmful. Sharp corners create cutting chi, called sha-chi. If your plot of ground is situated at the end of a cul-de-sac or neighbouring buildings have sharp corners that point at your property, a great deal of sha-chi may be arriving at your property. Use curved pathways and groups of trees and bushes (see p. 24) to protect yourself and your house from this negative cutting chi energy.

Views

A view of water is considered to be beneficial as long as the distance from the house is great enough (see p. 34) and the water is clean. If there is no view, strategic garden planning may create balance: small areas of water or running streams are relatively easy to build oneself. The visual impression of depth in your garden can be achieved through the skillful creation of pathways or by ensuring that tension is provided through including plants and bushes of different heights.

Yin and Yang

According to Chinese tradition, the entire universe is laid out on two basic complementary principles called yin and yang. These two principles always occur in pairs and ensure harmony and equilibrium. They should be present in balanced ratios on your plot of ground, where shady and sunny, damp and dry areas, lower lying and raised areas, tall and short plants, curved and geometric forms as well as quiet and active zones can be found. If yin and yang are not in equilibrium in your garden, it can cause disharmony in your life. Feng shui techniques will have a balancing effect here, too.

Choice of plants

When choosing plants, you should also consider the existing factors of light, warmth, moisture, wind and soil on site. If you choose indigenous plants that are suited to the growing conditions, your garden will be fairly low-maintenance.

Your garden and the law

Before planting new things, find out something about the planning rules in your area, such as the minimum distance of trees and bushes from your boundaries. This will also depend on the heights of the trees or bushes. It will vary depending on the county or state and your local authority should be able to give you the information you need.

What you want to achieve

You cannot see beneficial feng shui – you feel it! The ideal garden will fit naturally into the surrounding landscape so it does not appear out of place. Anyone coming into your garden or looking at it from a distance will sense its inner harmony and be uplifted by it. It is like dipping into a spring that dispenses energy and regenerating powers. Instead of seeing just one detail, the garden lover and owner of a feng shui garden will look at the effects of the garden as a whole. In this way, the whole garden will become a map of the gardener's personality and will present you with refreshing new details wherever you walk.

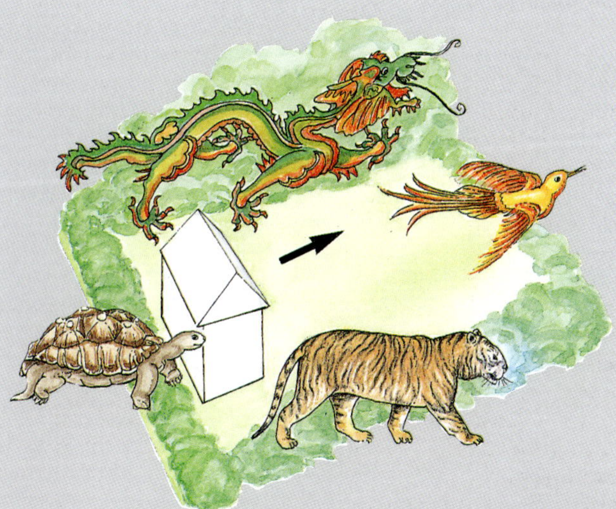

The four heavenly animals

The surroundings of a house are described by feng shui masters using four mythological symbols.

- The back of the house (seen from the main viewing direction, see arrow in the illustration) should be secure and protected. This is where we find the Tortoise that reliably protects our back with its strong shell.
- At the front of the house, however, the view should be wide and uninterrupted. This is symbolised by the mythical Phoenix bird that flies up high into the sky and can see far across the landscape.
- On the left side of the garden we find the active and dominant Dragon who is the mighty guardian of the house.
- On the right side of the garden we have the Tiger. He is more gentle and lower than the dragon but always ready to react to any threat.

Make sure there is an harmonious relationship between the four heavenly animals in your garden. There are more details of how to put this into practice over the page.

Your garden and its surroundings

Before you actually start designing and planning your garden, you should think seriously about the land you have, its surroundings and the existing features and conditions of the site.

Shape of the garden

Illustration 1

The shape of the garden should ideally be square or rectangular so that the outside world does not protrude into your personal life space.

L-shaped plots. The ideal solution would be to buy the missing portion of land to make up the full rectangle but, of course, this is not often possible. The simplest alternative is to break up and soften the effect through a more fluid style of planting along the boundary, for example, with an open hedge.

Triangular plots. These produce a very attractive and fiery energy (see p. 20) that often shows itself in the particularly hot temperaments of the inhabitants. Here you can either use a water feature to soften the triangular shape or provide a balance in the following way: divide up the plot in mainly trapezoid zones, by extending and completing the lines of the house walls, for example as paths, beds or low hedges. A traditional feng shui solution is to bury a red cord along these lines.

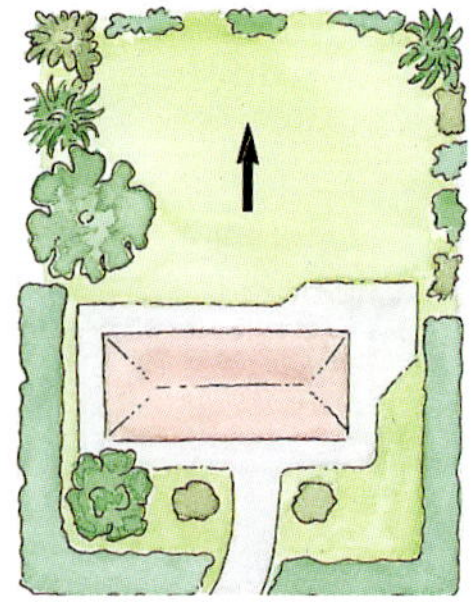

***2** Armchair principle: Safety and security.*

The armchair principle

Illustration 2

The garden should correspond to the classic four heavenly animals (see p. 11), a more modern term for this being 'the armchair principle'. The meaning of the term is that it is a place where we feel particularly at ease in our surroundings, where we are protected at our backs and on both sides, and where we can enjoy a wide, uninterrupted view.

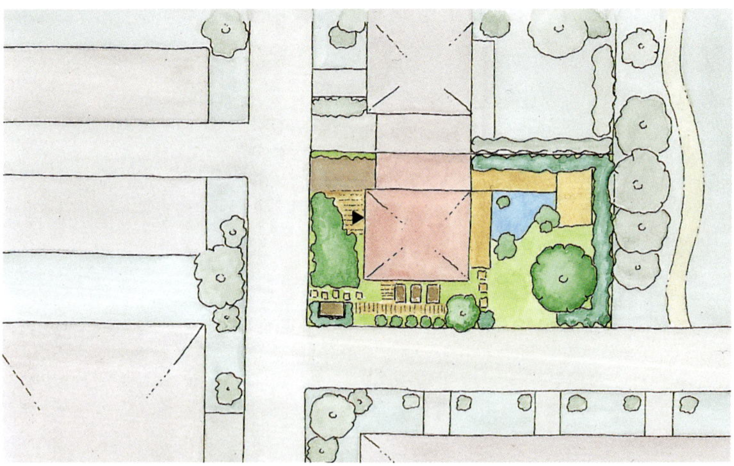

***1** Regularly shaped gardens provide the best conditions for an harmonious garden with supportive chi.*

This should feel just like sitting in an armchair with a comfortable backrest, armrests on the sides and a good view in front of you. At the back of the house, for example, an open hedge will provide protection. The main garden on the Phoenix side on the other hand, should be designed in an open manner. In gardens without a proper view, it is recommended to create a small Phoenix here in the form of a low mound of earth (see illustration 3). Where there is a pleasant view, however, the Phoenix may be represented by a neighbour's tree or a hill on the horizon. On the left-hand Dragon side, the plants or the neighbouring surroundings should be larger and more dynamic; on the right, the Tiger side, they should be lower, rounder and more flowing. If there is a reversal of this, and the left side is weaker and the right side stronger, you may be able to strengthen the Dragon side with careful planting. If there is no room there to add large plants, you may be able to create a symbolic Dragon in the form of a rugged rock with sharp edges and corners. The Tiger, on the other hand, can be emphasised with soft and round shaped objects and features.

A beautiful view from your window

Illustrations 3 and 4

Quite often, the surroundings outside the garden boundaries are not particularly inviting or harmonious. Factories, fire walls, multi-storey buildings, streets, shopping centres and so on all create ugly views and constantly have an energy-draining effect. In these cases, it is even more important to aim for an harmonious view from your window. Plant your own green screens in front of these ugly views and make use of attractive accessories. If there is enough space, you can plant an open hedge in the background. Climbing plants provide a screen in small spaces and will cover walls, fences and espaliers with greenery.

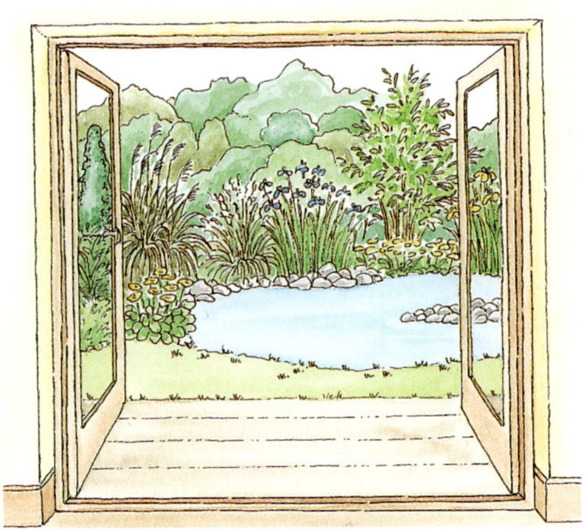

***3** The Phoenix can be represented by a bush or a low mound of earth.*

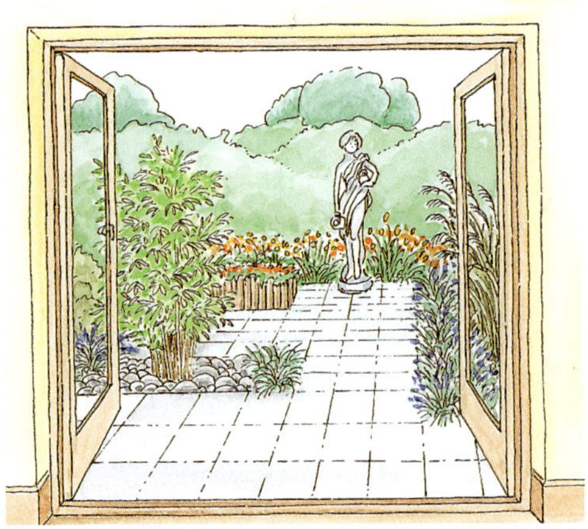

***4** Ugly views are cleverly disguised with plants and accessories in this garden.*

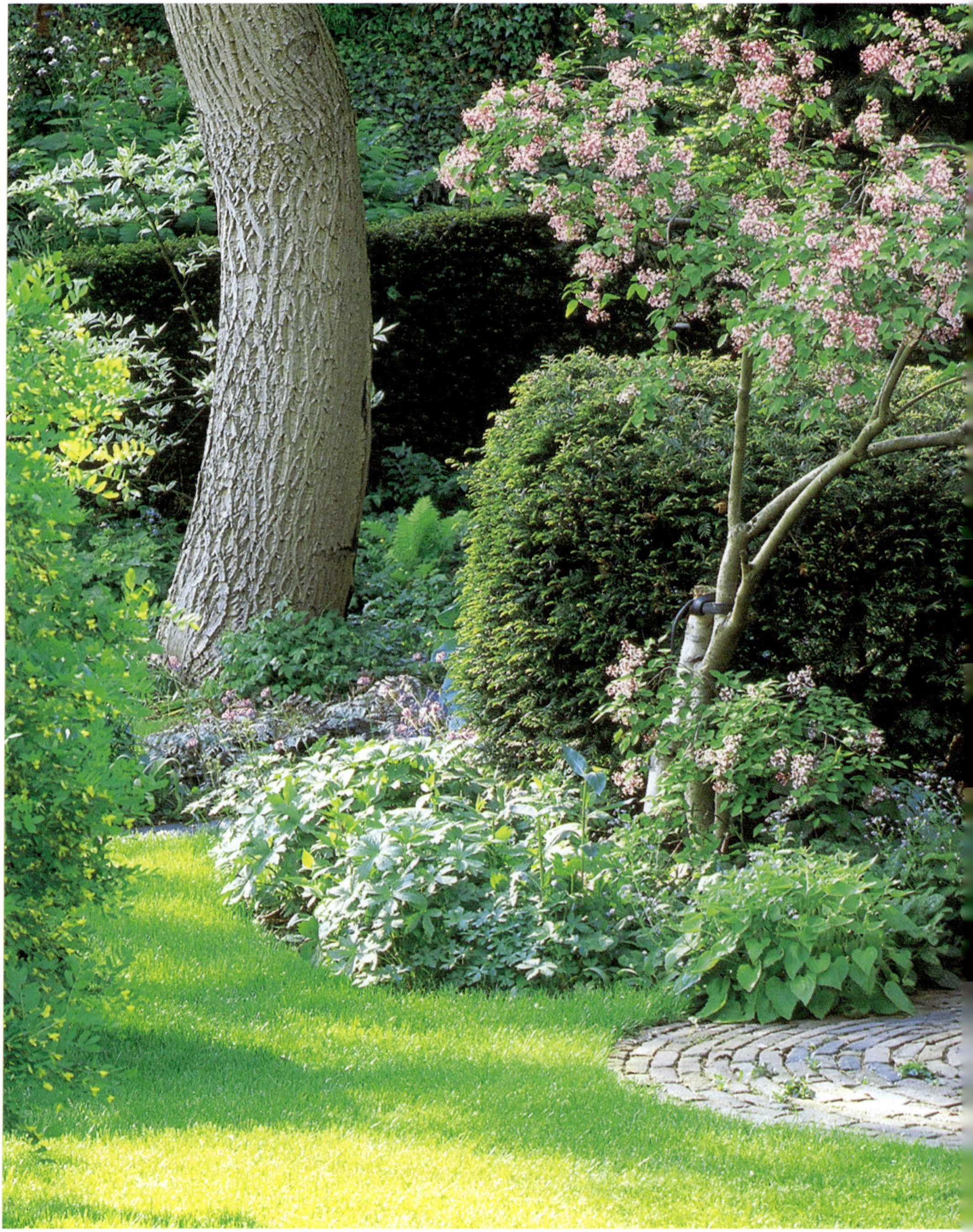

Feng Shui techniques

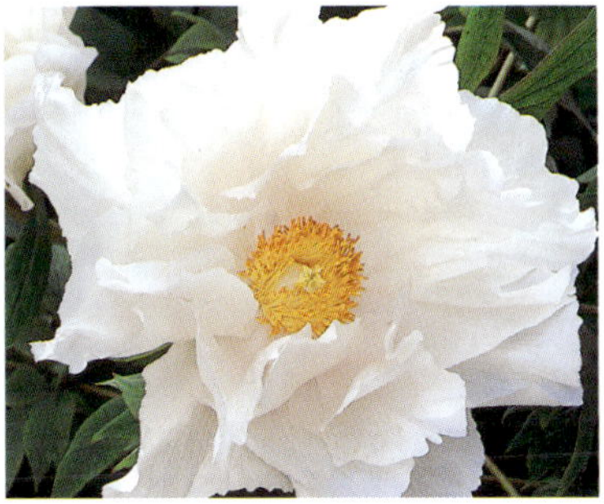

A bush peony (Paeonia hybrid) can enhance energy.

The teaching of feng shui offers various means of exploring the energy flow in your garden and can, if necessary, be used to enhance the energy.

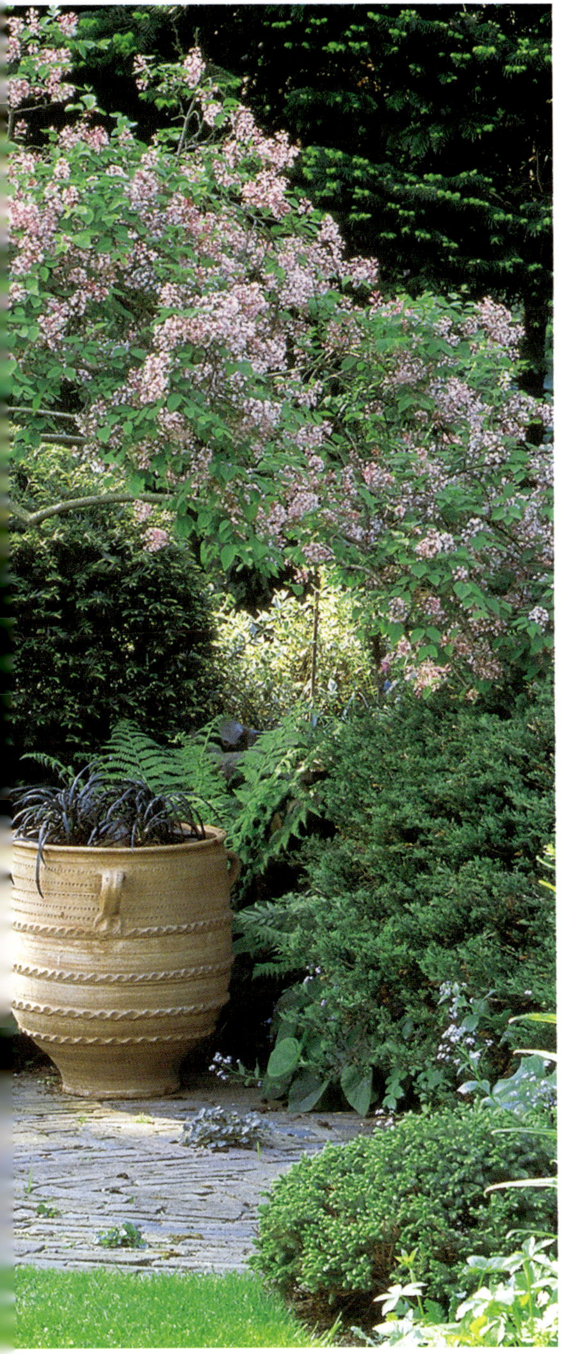

Terracotta pots and bricks fortify the Earth energies and associated bagua zones.

Feng shui techniques

The bagua

The bagua (see pull-out sheet, opposite) is a very helpful device for the correct planning of a feng shui garden. The word bagua means literally 'the body of the dragon'. If you imagine your garden as the body of the dragon it makes it easier to understand how the nine bagua fields can be put to use. Every part of the bagua symbolises a particular area of your life and everything you experience in your life is connected with you on an invisible plane. Even your garden is a part of your own field and as such is capable of expressing a part of you. You will be surprised, when you look at things through feng shui eyes, how your view will illuminate the various events and situations in your life. Look upon your own surrounding field as a mirror of your personality and recognise that in all things there are great opportunities for change.
Above all, have lots of fun with your discoveries!

Career

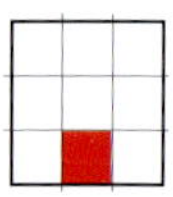

This area or field of the garden represents the flow of your life and shows how close you really are to your destiny in your professional as well as private life. For this reason, this area should should convey a flowing appearance through planting design, pathways or shapes in the terrain.

Partnership

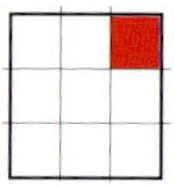

This bagua zone provides information on your relationship not only with your partner but also with your friends, colleagues and neighbours. It is a particularly sensitive area and can often even forewarn you: if plants in this zone begin to become sickly you should immediately pay a lot of time and attention to interpersonal relationships. You will be able to read your success from the condition of your plants.

Family

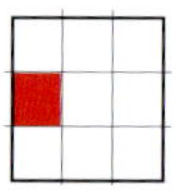

This part of the garden mirrors your own family background, that is your roots and your relationship to your parents, ancestors and also to your superiors and authority figures. As this part of the garden also represents the past, many difficulties in realising new ideas can often be removed by attending to weak spots in the family zone and by encouraging positive energy in this area of the garden. Incidentally, unresolved problems can often block the chi in this zone, so it is worth clearing up the garden from scratch, removing tree stumps and sickly plants.

Wealth

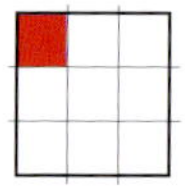

This zone points to the potential of your own spiritual and material wealth. It also symbolises your ability to recognise the true values of life, to accept them and to appreciate them.

Centre (Tai chi)

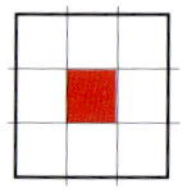

The centre represents your life energy and also your health. The more open and harmonious this very important area is, the more healing and centred vibrations will radiate outwards from the centre.

Helpful people

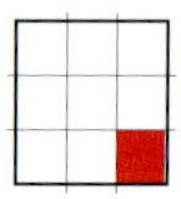

This area stands for support, help and protection. Whenever we are given exactly the kind of help that we need or seem to receive the information we require at exactly the right moment, this energy zone is being activated.

The bagua for your plot of ground

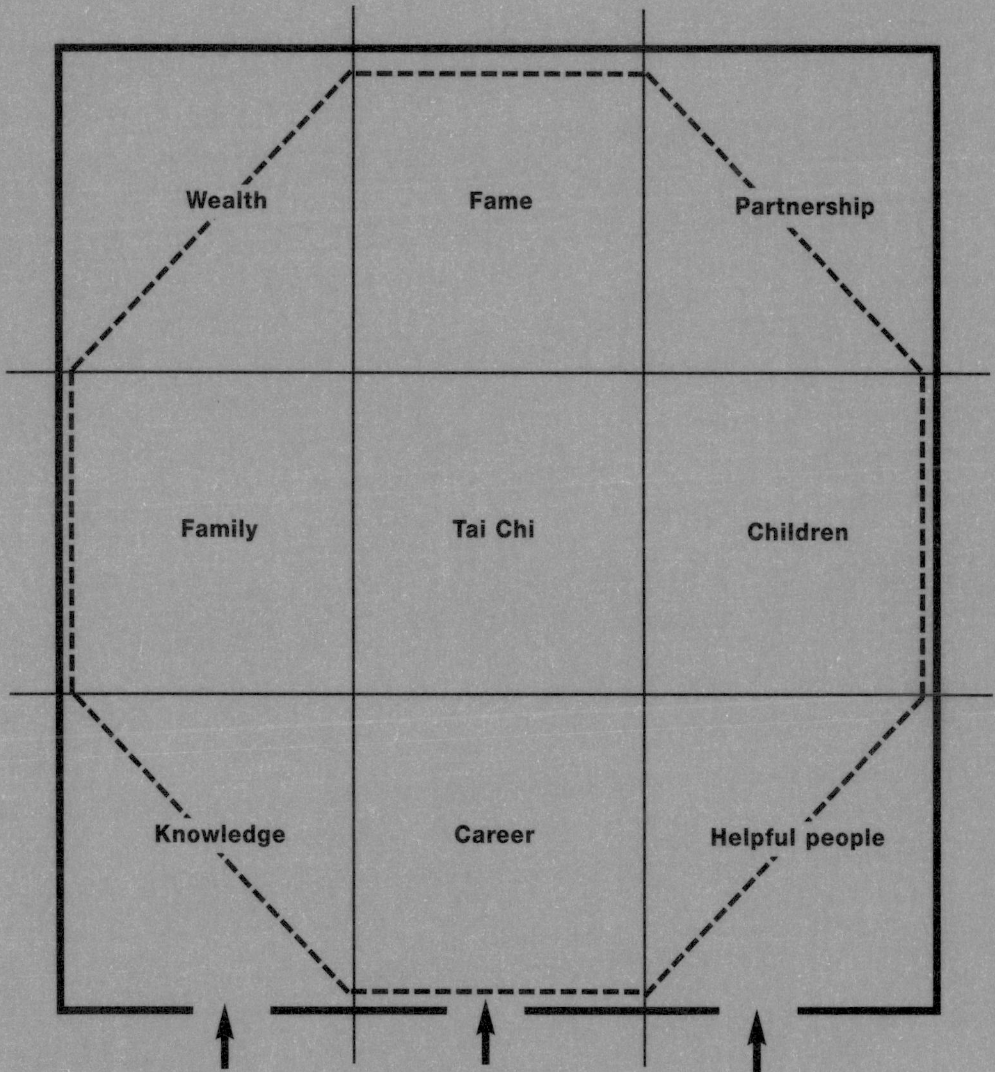

3 possible main entrances to the plot of ground

The bagua for your plot of ground

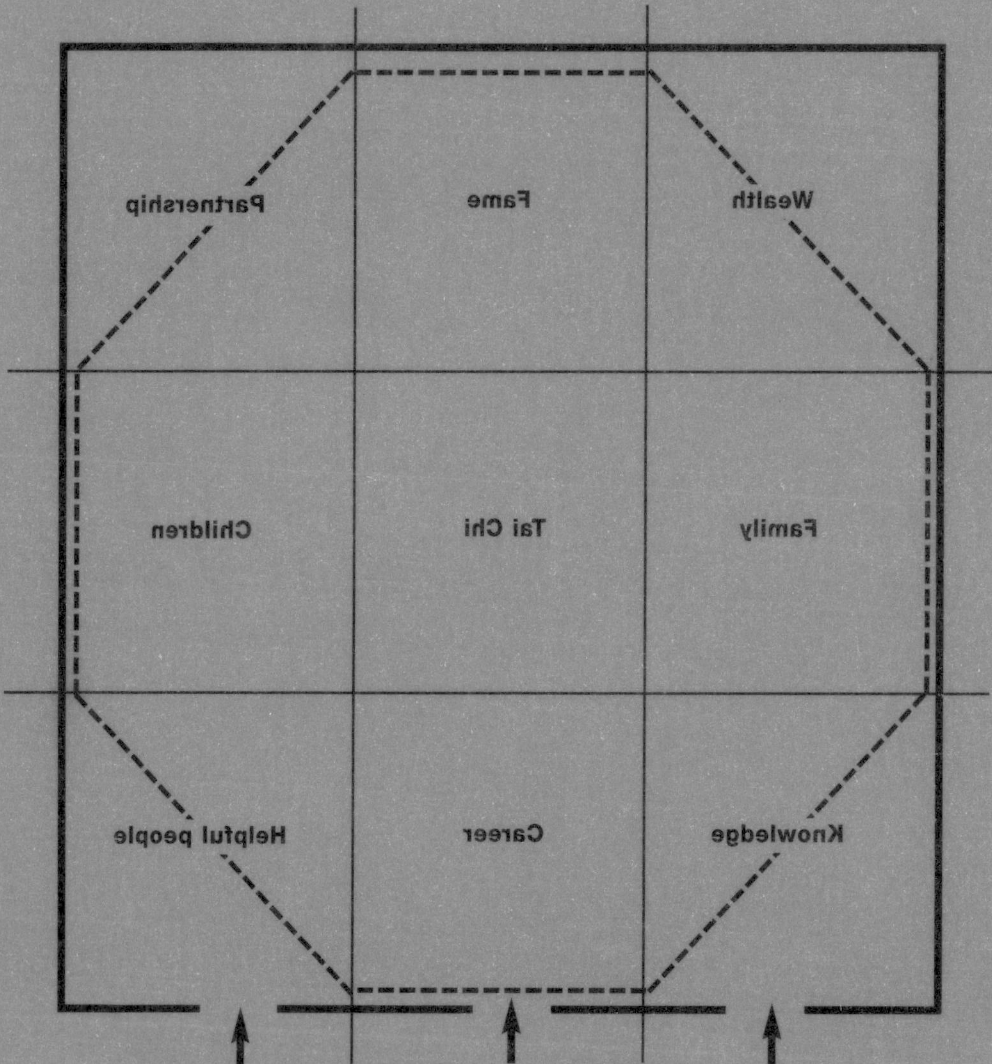

3 possible main entrances to the plot of ground

Children

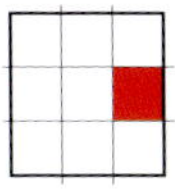

This zone is the most active and creativity-enhancing area of the garden. It provides information not only about your relationships with children in general, but also about how creative you are. If you are suffering from a lack of ideas, you should give a lot of attention to this part of the garden.

Knowledge

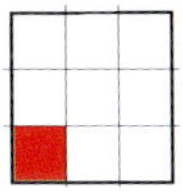

This part of the garden relates to your gift of intuition and your access to higher knowledge. This part of the garden should be a zone dedicated to peace and contemplation. This is where you can switch off particularly easily from everyday stress.

Fame

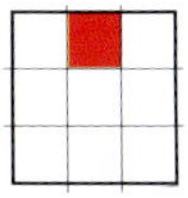

Your inner maturity and the outer radiation of the light of your personality are shown in this area. This is also where your public reputation is mirrored, reflecting how you are seen by the outside world.

The flow of energy in your garden

The life energy of chi is able to flow in soft currents on this property, actively supported by a free, open main entrance. A boundary of openly planted trees and bushes keeps the energy in the garden. All paths run in natural waves as the chi would be too concentrated and excessive on straight paths. Depending on the individual zone, the flow of energy enhances certain areas of life. You can find out which they are by placing the bagua grid over this plan (see following pages).

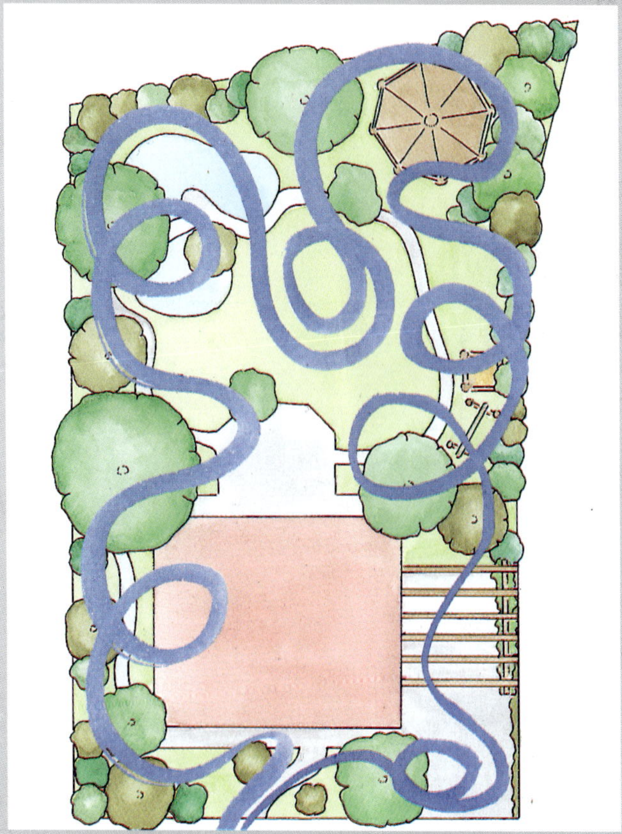

Using the bagua

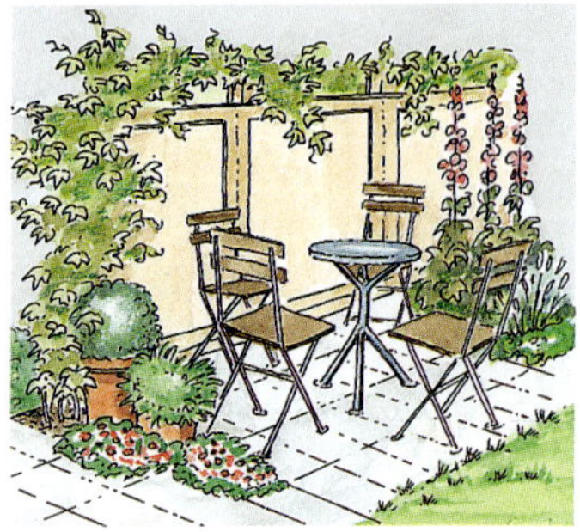

2 *A cosy sitting corner works well in the bagua zones of Family and Helpful People.*

The bagua is extremely easy to use: to begin with you should sketch a plan of your garden. A rectangular plot is ideal, but if yours is an irregular shape you can overcome this by sketching a closed rectangular shape over the top of your plan.

Extensions and deficient areas

There are many different ways in which a garden may deviate from the ideal shape:

- An extension exists if a few small areas (see illustration 1) jut out beyond the basic ideal shape. They may lie outside the bagua grid and tend to enhance the zones of which they are extensions. Consider them as particularly supportive as they point to your – perhaps undiscovered – strengths.
- A deficient area exists if the missing area is at least 50 per cent of the main area (measured by length or breadth). This is the case for many L-shaped gardens. The missing zones should be incorporated into the bagua. If one bagua zone is very much smaller than the rest there is likely to be a weakness in this area of your life, too. There are steps you can take to help balance this deficiency, however (see p. 48).
- One or several of the bagua fields may be enhanced by the house itself, perhaps because they are entirely enclosed by the building. This is often the case in small terraced houses with gardens. It is also an indication that these areas are particularly important for the people living in the house. No special measures will need to be introduced.

Constructing the bagua in the correct way

Illustration 1

If the proportions of the removable bagua plan do not coincide with your plot of ground, you will need to draw a rectangular sketch of your garden. Next, divide the four sides by three and connect the points you have found with horizontal and vertical lines. By doing this you will have sketched in the nine bagua fields exactly.

Important: The bagua should always be laid out so that the fields of Knowledge, Career and Helpful people are situated on the same side of the garden as the main entrance to the property.

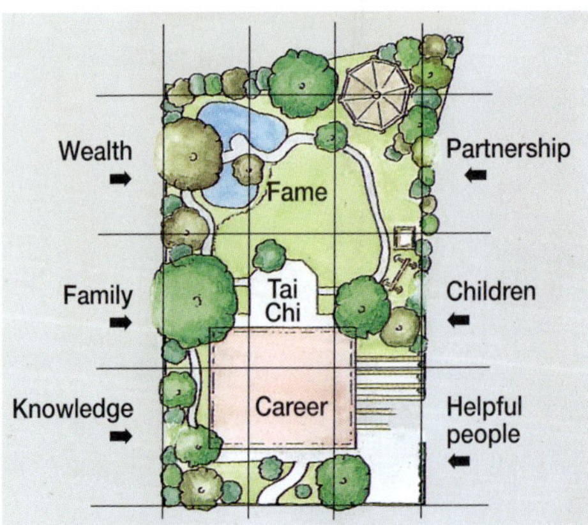

1 *The bagua zones were drawn into a plan of the plot of ground and show several extensions.*

Garden elements according to the bagua

Illustrations 2 to 7

Here are a few typical garden elements for the individual bagua zones (see p.16). Many more ideas and tips can be found starting on p. 50.

Family
A sitting place in a comfortable corner, with space for all the family is particularly good here (see illustration 2).

Helpful people
This is a good place for a sitting corner (see illustration 2) where you can get together with your friends.

Fame
Handsome accessories like a sculpture (see illustration 3) would be in the ideal position here and enhance the radiation of the field.

Centre (Tai chi)
The centre of the garden should represent a collecting place for the energy. Sculptures or figures with a special radiative energy (see illustration 3), or simply an open area, are ideal.

Knowledge
A peaceful, convex or protected cave-like sitting place is particularly good for this field (see illustration 4).

Partnership
This area should be designed in a particularly harmonious way. An intimate little pavilion to encourage relationships would be ideal (see illustration 5).

Career
This zone symbolises the flow of life, so running water, like this spring stone (see illustration 6), or even a simple bird bath, is very suitable in this field.

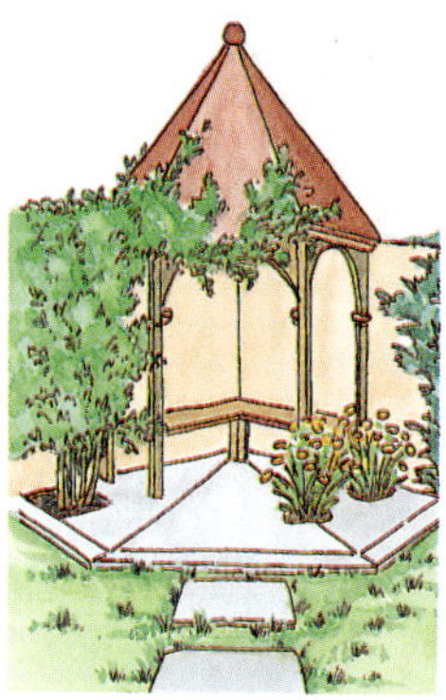

5 *An open pavilion for the Partnership zone.*

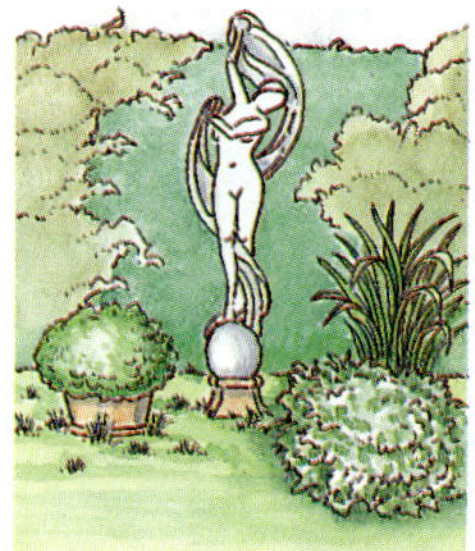

3 *Sculpted figures for Fame and the Centre.*

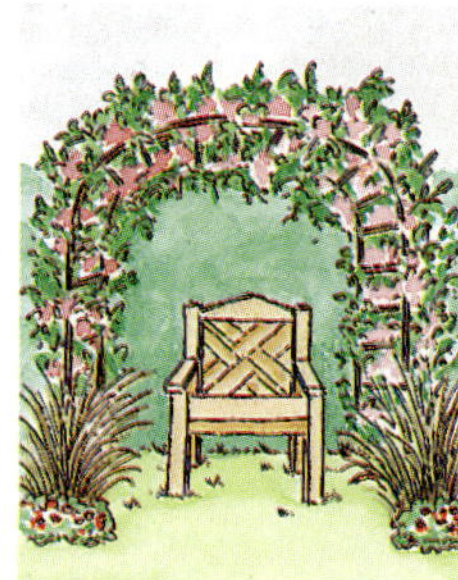

4 *A quiet place for Knowledge.*

Wealth
Water is associated with wealth, so running water in the shape of a spring stone would also be suitable in this area (see illustration 6).

Children
If you have children of your own, their sand pit, swings and play area are probably best situated in this area (see illustration 7).

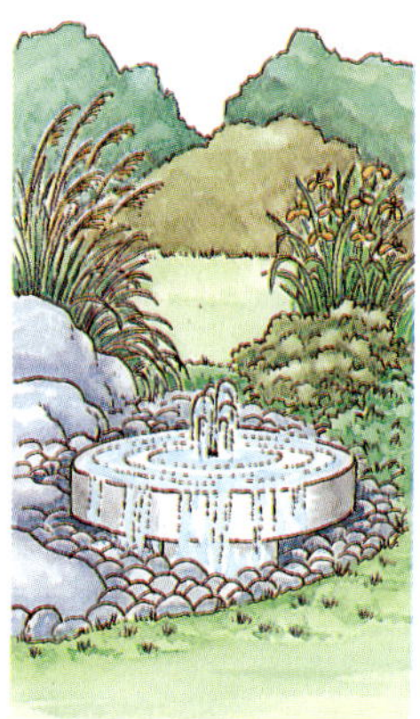

6 *Water for Career and Wealth.*

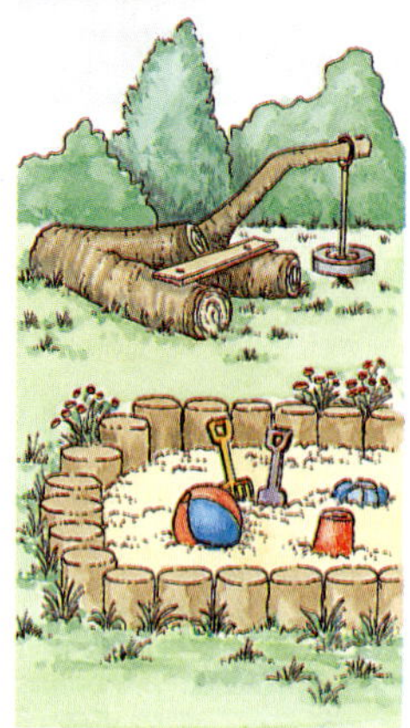

7 *A play area for Children.*

The five elements

The feng shui teaching of the five elements is based on five basic energy qualities and can be transferred to Western thinking:

- Wood symbolises energies that move upwards in a strong, slender ray.
- Fire stands for energies that run upwards in a point, like a triangle.
- Earth creates energies that work and move sideways and downwards.
- Metal rules energies that are condensed in a round shape and contract inwards.
- Water represents energies that spread irregularly, in waves.

When you consider the five elements of feng shui in this way, you will start to see your garden in a completely new light. The elements may also influence each other. Their relationships are in a constant state of flux and the five feng shui elements are often referred to as the five phases of change.

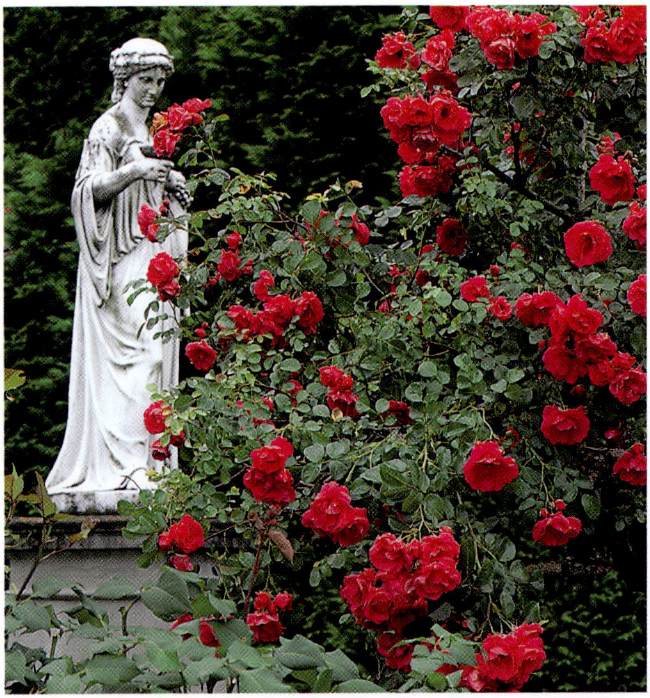

Accessories and plants concentrate the energies in your garden.

The two cycles

The supportive cycle of creation runs as follows: Wood supports Fire as it nourishes fire. Fire supports Earth by producing ash. Earth supports Metal as it contains ore. Metal supports Water as molten metal also flows. Water supports Wood by nourishing it.

When you are designing a garden it is important that every part of it should include these supportive conditions, as they in turn will nourish the general complement of energies.

The second cycle is the braking or inhibiting cycle of control. Wood inhibits Earth as it withdraws nutrients from it. Earth inhibits Water by forming boundaries to its free-flowing nature. Water inhibits Fire as it extinguishes flames. Fire inhibits Metal as it melts it. Metal inhibits Wood because the axe splits it.

The table on the right provides details of the five elements and the zones assigned to the bagua. The supportive and inhibiting energies, suitable shapes, colours, plants and accessories are also included. By following those guidelines you will be able to enhance or inhibit the different bagua zones effectively and balance them. Find out more about this on the following pages.

Element	Wood	Fire	Earth	Metal	Water
Associated bagua zone	Family, Wealth	Fame	Partnership, Knowledge, Centre	Children, Helpful people	Career
Supported by	Water (nourishes wood)	Wood (nourishes fire)	Fire (creates ash, that turns to earth)	Earth (contains metal ores)	Metal (molten metal flows like water)
Inhibited by	Metal (the axe splits wood)	Water (extinguishes fire)	Wood (obtains nutrients from the earth)	Fire (melts the metal)	Earth (forms boundaries for water)
Landscape/ surrounding shapes	slender tree, masts, tower	pointed hill, gable of house	flat landscape, flat roof	round hill, domed roof	wavy hills or mounds, irregularly shaped roofs
Associated colours	green, light blue to violet blue	red, wine-red to lilac red, pink	yellow, orange, brown	white, silver, gold	black, dark blue
Plant shapes	tall, upward growth, column-shaped, climbing	objects that point upwards, pointed leaves, thorns, prickles	low, spreading growth, directed towards the earth	spherical, round to semi-round growth	wavy leaves and shoots, irregular growth
Typical plants	juniper (*Juniperus communis* 'Hibernica'), Yew (*Taxus baccata* 'Fastigiata' toxic), clematis, mullein (*Verbascum phoeniceum*)	(*Picea glauca* 'Conica', berberis (*Berberis thunbergii atropurpurea*), roses (*Rosa* species), red hot pokers (*Kniphofia* hybrids), bush peony (*Paeonia* hybrids)	juniper (*Juniperus communis* 'Repanda'), broom (*Genista lydia*), honeysuckle (*Lonicera pileata*, toxic), alyssum (*Alyssum saxatile*), stonecrop (*Sedum acre,* toxic), throatwort (*Uvularia grandiflora*)	box tree cut spherically (*Buxus sempervirens*, toxic), Balsam fir (*Abies balsamea* 'Nana'), mountain avens (*Dryas octopetala*), gypsophila	*Cotoneaster adpressus,* Hinoki cypress (*Chamaecyparis obtusa),* Cobnut (*Corylus avellana* 'Contorta'), hosta species, water plants
Accessories associated with the element	columns or pillars, posts, tall objects	garden torches, modern garden art, barbecues, fireplace	figures, sculptures, pots and surfaces of clay, ground covering of gravel or stone	gazing balls and other spherical objects, tables, arches	water, standing or running, bird baths, wind chimes

Using the five elements

You will be able to make simple improvements in the individual areas of the garden with the help of the table (see p. 21) and the bagua (see pp. 18 and 19). The illustrations on the right will also provide you with an overview of the elements you can use.

Checking every bagua field

Supposing you would like to check the Partnership field in your garden. Start by looking in the fourth column of the table. You will find the word under the element Earth to which it has been assigned. This means that all colours, shapes, plants and accessories that correspond to the element Earth are well suited to activate the Partnership zone. The lower four sections of the Earth column give a general summary of the features you might wish to include.

The Partnership zone will also be supported by everything that corresponds to the element Fire, as you will be able to see in the third column.

Important: Also check whether inhibiting factors are present in the zone. In our example, that would be everything assigned to the element Wood, as shown in the first column. If you notice an excess of something, you can restore the balance in one of the following ways:

- Activate and encourage the Partnership zone as described above.
- Place something beside the inhibiting feature that is assigned to the element Metal, and that, in turn, will inhibit the element Wood. For example, plant box tree spheres around a column-shaped juniper bush.
- You could transplant the unwanted woody plants or woody accessories into a zone where they would enhance the effect. In our example this would be the field of Fame.
- If the supporting element Fire is being inhibited by a lot of water you will need to take the same approach.

Assigning plants to the elements

With the help of the table and some good plant catalogues or reference books, you will soon learn how to assign individual plants to the elements according to their growth and colours. You will also discover that elements occur in pairs in many species. Generally, one is more dominant and the other weaker. There will also be seasonal changes, for example, at flowering time. Think about which characteristic of the species dominates for the longest time or is most conspicuous and then assign it to the corresponding element.

Wood

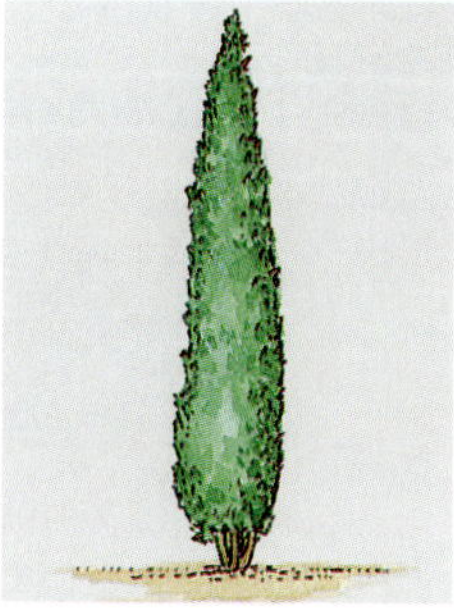

1 *Wood plant: Juniper.*

Plants: All species and varieties that are slender, column-shaped and grow tall or climb should be assigned to the element Wood.
Colours: Green, light to mid-blue, blue violet.
Accessories: All objects that rise up tall, are slim or slender, including objects made of wood.

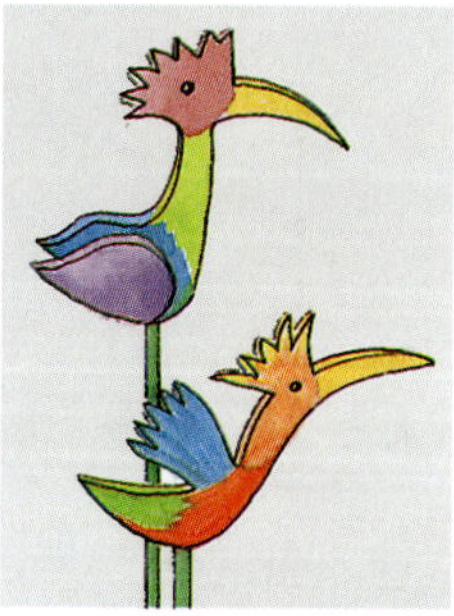

2 *Wood accessories: wooden birds.*

Fire

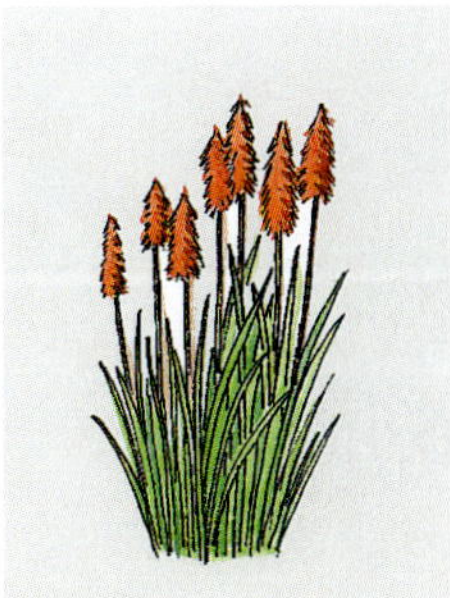

3 *Fire plant: red hot poker.*

Plants: All species and varieties that grow upwards into a point and/or that have pointed or lance-shaped leaves, prickles or thorns.
Colours: red, wine red, purple red, pink.
Accessories: Garden lighting, barbecues or fireplaces, modern garden art.

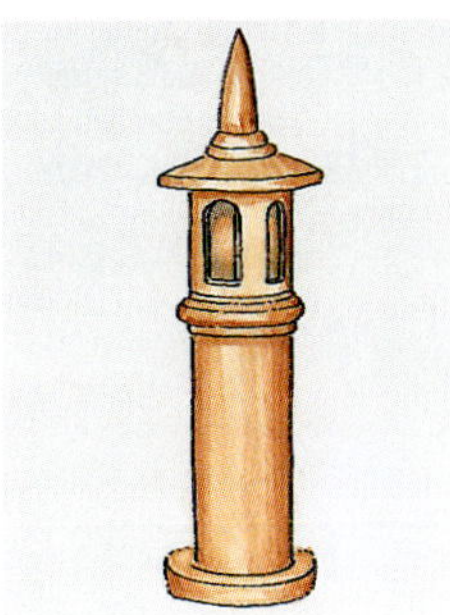

4 *Fire accessory: garden lamp.*

Earth

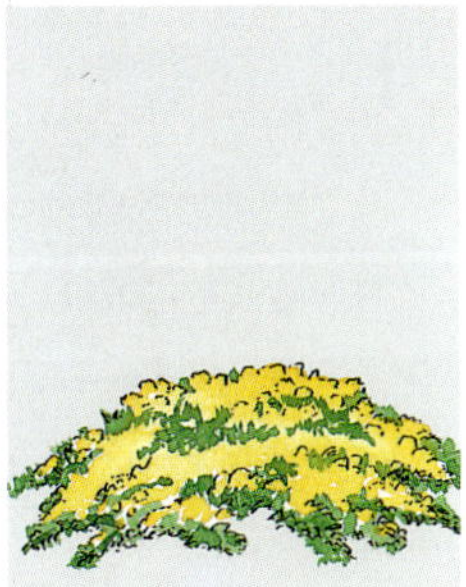

5 *Earth plant: Alyssum.*

Plants: All that grow low and spread out regularly, also ground-cover plants. All species whose branches and/or leaves point towards the ground.
Colours: yellow, orange, brown.
Accessories: Figures, pots, surfaces made of clay, stone or gravel, brick or stone walls.

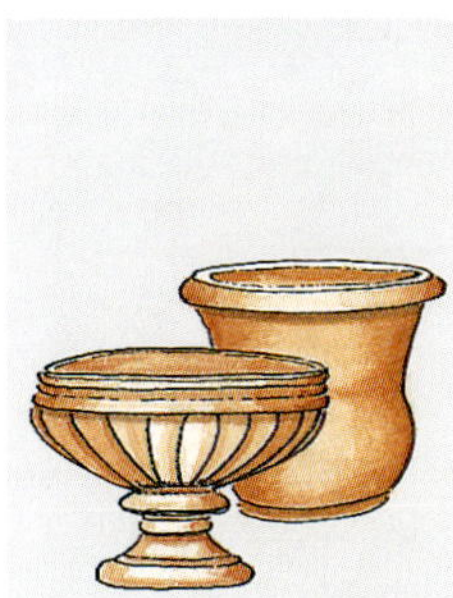

6 *Earth accessories: terracotta pots.*

Metal

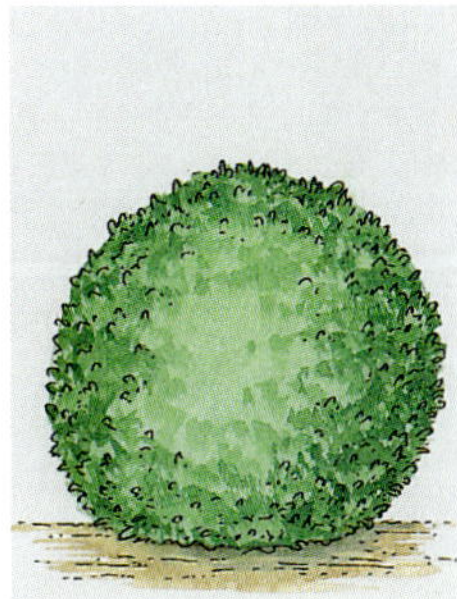

7 *Metal plant: spherical box tree.*

Plants: All plants that are left to grow naturally, or are cut into a spherical shape, or have a semi-rounded or rounded growth.
Colours: white, silver, gold.
Accessories: Everything with rounded shapes – gazing balls, arches, round tables, flower-beds and stones.

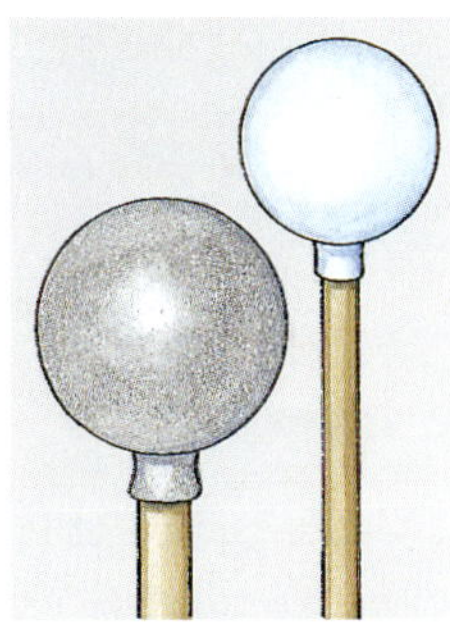

8 *Metal accessories: gazing balls of all sizes.*

Water

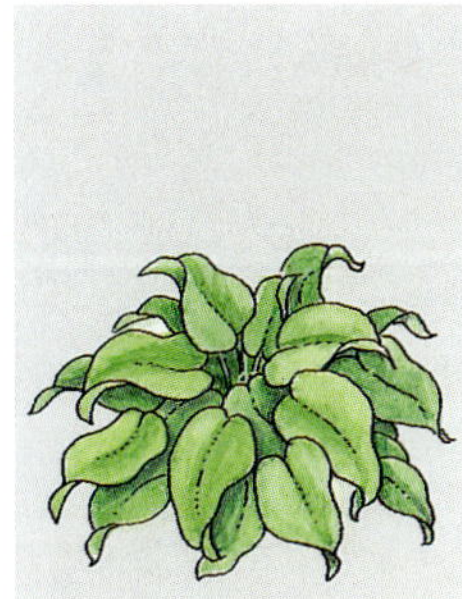

9 *Water plant: wavy-leafed hosta.*

Plants: All species and varieties with wavy leaves and/or shoots. Irregular growth.
Colours: black, dark blue.
Accessories: Running or standing water such as a stream, spring stone, pond or bird bath, wind chimes.

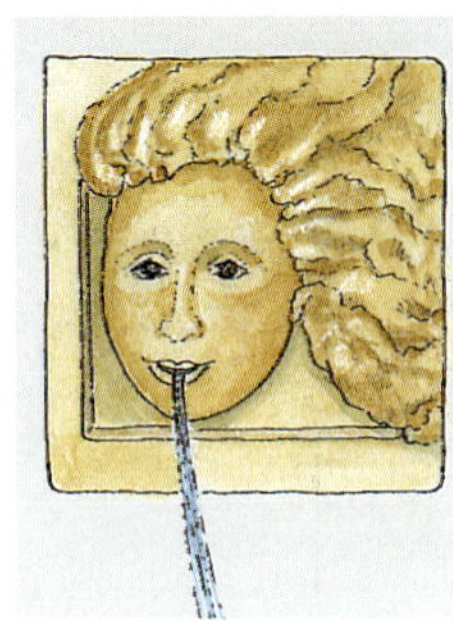

10 *Water accessory: running water.*

Your surroundings

Man has always attached great importance to his surroundings, believing them to hold special powers. Until quite recently, the gnarled old tree in the heart of the village really was a focal point for village life and was often thought to have special, beneficial powers. Today, our surroundings have changed radically and it is not at all rare for bad influences to predominate. The questions on the right will help you to recognise which disturbing influences should be removed.

You've identified the problem, what next?

Once you've worked through the questionnaire you will realise that all questions to which the answer is yes require some kind of action.
Sha-chi (see p. 10) should be braked or transformed if sharp corners are in a direct line with your house or garden seating areas. Depending on the height of the source, this can be overcome by planting trees or bushes to deflect the sha-chi.
In the case of low-lying sources of disturbance, such as roads, you should avoid any kind of direct connection by a path to the house and construct a path that curves generously and will inhibit the chi energy.
Drive gazing balls on posts into

Your surroundings	**Yes**	**No**
Sha-chi sources in your surroundings		
Does a road run straight towards your garden or, worse, is it situated at the end of a cul-de-sac?	☐	☐
Is your garden situated in the curve of a sharp bend or, worse, at the end of a hairpin bend?	☐	☐
Is your garden situated on a hill where it is completely exposed with no protection from wind and weather?	☐	☐
Is your garden situated in a cup-shaped hollow, in which everything is collected and stored up?	☐	☐
Does your garden border on buildings with sharp corners on walls or roofs?	☐	☐
Is there a canal with dirty, cloudy water beside your property?	☐	☐
In the surroundings of your property, are there very few green areas or gardens, but lots of masts or tall street lamps?	☐	☐
Do you sense that the surroundings of your house are unbalanced and inharmonious?	☐	☐
Is the street outside your house very noisy, or are there other sources of disturbance and unrest like public houses or factories?	☐	☐
Do the neighbouring buildings have strongly varying heights and restless shapes?	☐	☐
Does a steep hill or a tall building block your view?	☐	☐
Access for people and chi		
Is the garden surrounded with a dense, visually impenetrable hedge on all sides?	☐	☐
Is the entrance gate difficult to find and/or open?	☐	☐
Is the rubbish bin is placed in such a way that it is the first thing a visitor would see?	☐	☐
Is your drive straight and does it run directly towards the house or garage?	☐	☐

Your surroundings	Yes	No
Does the path to the house run straight and/or directly towards the entrance door?	☐	☐
Are the entrance area and the entrance to the house badly lit?	☐	☐
Along the path to the door, do plants, trees and branches protrude onto the path?	☐	☐
Are there loose flagstones in the path or are there holes in the surface?	☐	☐
Does the front garden look forlorn, uninteresting, unwelcoming or badly kept?	☐	☐
Are you unable to find the Tortoise, the Phoenix, the Dragon or the Tiger in your garden?	☐	☐
The garden itself, chi's arena		
Is the view into the garden blocked by a dense tangled mass of bushes or trees?	☐	☐
Is the focal point of the garden a decaying summerhouse, a grey wall or other large structure?	☐	☐
Are there any dead trees or even rubbish lying about in the garden?	☐	☐
Is the garden fairly empty and dominated by a low-maintenance lawn?	☐	☐
Are such relaxing elements as water, figures, stones, lamps or rose arches missing almost entirely from the garden?	☐	☐
Is there a steep, non-terraced slope in the garden?	☐	☐
Is the compost heap untidy or situated in the bagua zone of Wealth?	☐	☐
Are you tackling pests like slugs and snails or diseases like mildew with strong chemical pesticides and fungicides?	☐	☐

the ground (see p. 48) or create a protective gateway, for example in the shape of a rose arch.
It works like a dividing element (see p. 36).

Good chi. The entrance should be clear and easily accessible for people and chi flowing in. However, avoid creating absolutely straight paths (see pp 10 and 36). Follow the principles of the four heavenly animals (see p. 11) and do a major tidy-up in the garden, concentrating on removing all blocking elements from the Centre (Tai chi). Ensure there is a balanced ratio between evergreen and deciduous species, and between green and flowering plants. Use suitable accessories (see p. 22) and find out how to deal with steep slopes (see p. 30).
Care. Do not disturb the harmony in your garden by employing chemicals for fertilising or the control of diseases and pests. Organic fortifying and protective plant extracts can be used instead (see p. 44).
You will also be able to supply the soil with nutrients through the use of green fertilisers (see p. 30) or compost (see p. 44). Do not build your compost heap in the Wealth field, but in another zone, as compost only represents future wealth.

Your own inner state

As you may have already read in the introduction to the bagua (see p. 16), every zone or field of the garden reflects a different aspect of your life. Before beginning to plan a feng shui garden you should not only meticulously study the surroundings, but also conduct a bit of an analysis of your own life to date. The questionnaire on the right is divided up according to the bagua zones. Take a few minutes to answer the questions, and try to be as objective and honest as possible with your answers.

What would you like to change?

You will soon notice that all the questions to which you answer 'no' mean you should improve the relevant aspects of your life. You will achieve this by using the bagua as described (see p. 18-19).
Supposing that by using the questionnaire you have discovered the most pressing problem at present is that relationships keep breaking up. This means you should take a look at the Partnership zone of your garden and at the table on p. 21. There you will see that this zone is governed by the element Earth, and supported by Fire and inhibited by Wood.

Your inner state	**Yes**	**No**
Career		
I am fairly satisfied with what I am doing and what I have achieved in my career.	☐	☐
The course of my life shows me that I have chosen the right path.	☐	☐
I can rely on my 'inner voice' and usually heed it.	☐	☐
Partnership		
I am considered to be easy to get along with and my career and business relationships run smoothly and harmoniously.	☐	☐
On the whole, I am living in a beautiful, happy and fulfilling love relationship.	☐	☐
My neighbours are nice people and we are always happy to see each other.	☐	☐
Family		
My parents like/liked coming to visit and we have/had a good relationship with each other.	☐	☐
My grandparents are/were my favourite advisors and are/were very important to me.	☐	☐
My relationships with superiors are good and they are always ready to listen to me.	☐	☐
Wealth		
I am quite content with the things life has to offer me.	☐	☐
My financial situation is balanced, even if I do not have great wealth.	☐	☐
I have quite a healthy sense of self and show it.	☐	☐
Centre		
I enjoy good health and and am very rarely ill.	☐	☐
I feel fairly centred, and am often filled with energy and get-up-and-go.	☐	☐

Your inner state	Yes	No
I am considered to be very balanced and do not allow myself to be upset very quickly.	☐	☐
Helpful people		
I am always surprised by how many good things seem to happen to me.	☐	☐
I am lucky enough to have a good friend with whom I can talk openly about everything.	☐	☐
If I am convinced that something is good and right I am happy to give it my full support.	☐	☐
Children		
If you have children: My children are doing well and my relationship with them is very balanced.	☐	☐
If you have no children: I like children very much and I am happy to have them around me.	☐	☐
I am very creative and I live out this potential in my everyday life and work.	☐	☐
Knowledge		
Other people regard me as very fond of learning and I find it easy to remember new information.	☐	☐
I give a lot of thought to the spiritual aspects of life.	☐	☐
My intuition is very reliable.	☐	☐
Fame		
Other people's opinions of me as a person are of little importance to me.	☐	☐
I make a conscious daily effort to improve and develop my personality.	☐	☐
My public reputation is good and I am well respected by other people.	☐	☐

Are there many slender woody plants like the column-shaped juniper (*Juniperus communis* 'Hibernica') growing there or any tall woody accessories like lamps or flagpoles that might be diverting energy from the Earth? In the case of inhibiting influences, proceed as described on p. 22. Activate the Partnership zone with the element Earth, such as with low-growing or ground-cover plants in shades of yellow, orange and brown and objects or ground coverings made of clay or stone. Enliven this zone by means of fiery shades of red, plants with pointed growth, garden lighting or modern sculptures. Tend this area of the garden particularly carefully. This conscious tender loving care and attention to the problem zones can create an energy boost that will help you to recognise new opportunities and use them properly. Check the other areas to see if you could make any improvements. In the case of zones that are missing altogether, make sure there is a balance as described on p. 48.

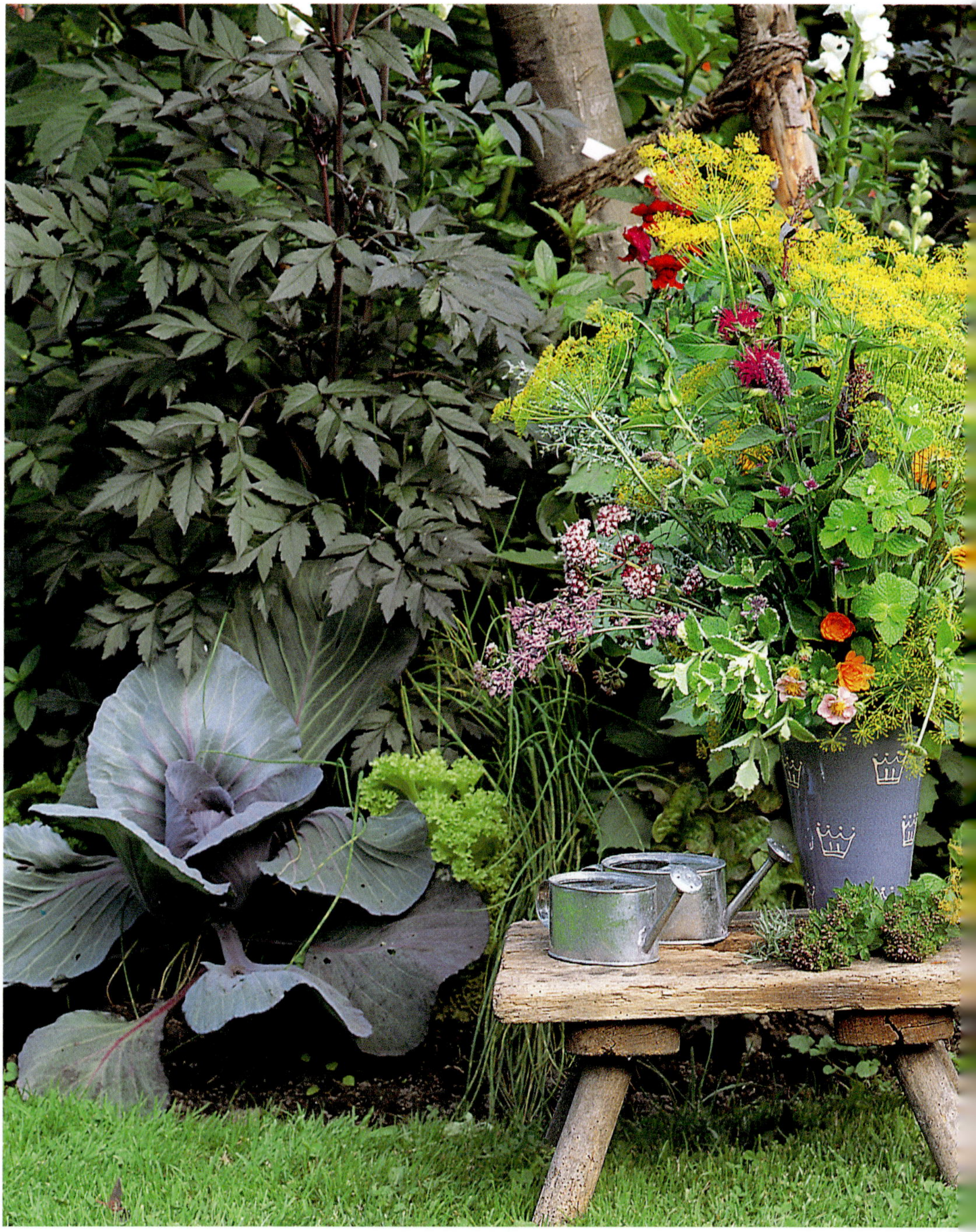

Planning and enjoying

A garden of the senses

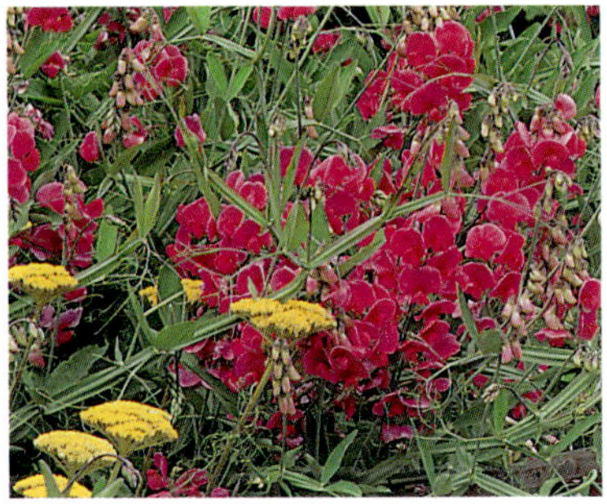

Scented sweet peas (Lathyrus odoratus) smell beautiful and can also provide a colourful screen.

There are a few basic rules when you are designing a feng shui garden from scratch and these apply when you are redesigning an existing garden, too. Above all, a feng shui garden should appeal to all five senses – this chapter is all about the sensual side of the garden.

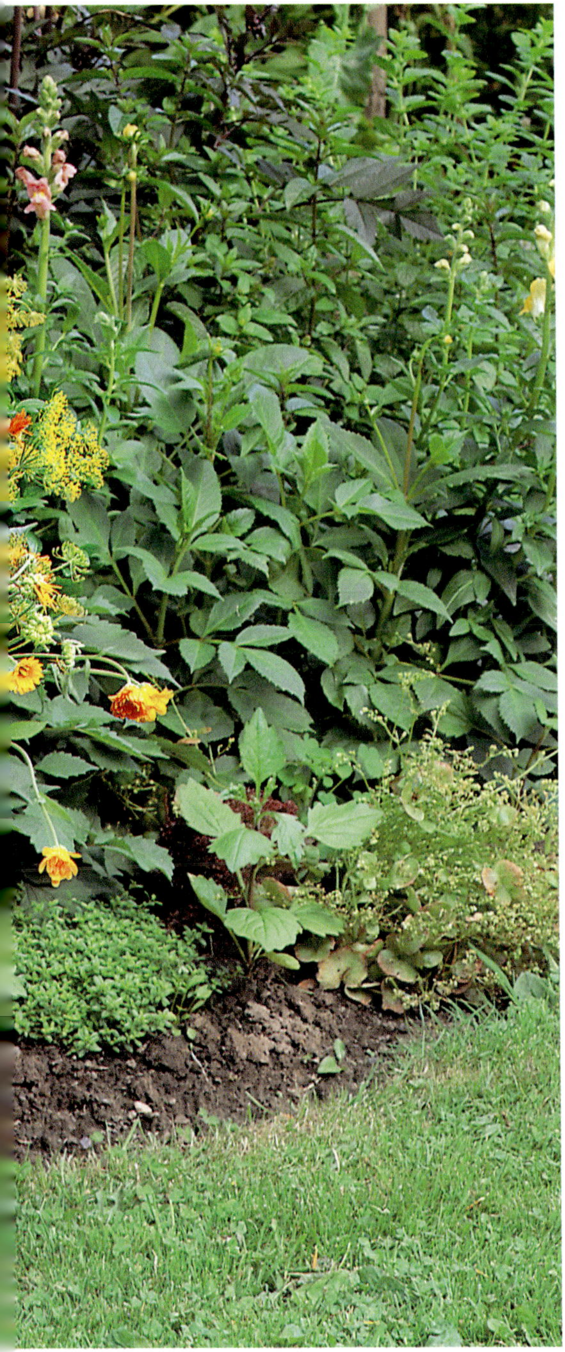

Herbs and vegetables are very important in a true garden of the senses.

The first steps

If you are planning to design a garden for the first time after building a new house, or if you are taking over a neglected garden, you should first dig the soil over and improve it.

Clearing. Inspect your plot of ground very carefully and remove all dead plants. Tree stumps should be dug out and all rubbish and debris should be collected and removed.

Green fertiliser. This is the most natural way of improving the quality of the soil. Depending on the species or mixture of seed, you can sow this from spring right through to the second month of autumn. You should be able to find seeds for this in most good garden centres. Among the standard green fertiliser plants are also some with attractive, scented flowers, like tansy (*Phacelia tanacetifolia)*, clover (*Trifolium incarnatum*) and nasturtium (*Tropaeolum majus*). The fully developed plants are cut, left lying for a few days and then worked loosely into the soil.

Get to know your garden. Give yourself some time to get to know this new piece of land. You may already have some trees, bushes and shrubs there. Walk around and ask yourself which plants appeal to you most, which ones you are indifferent to and which ones you actually dislike. Keep your eyes open when you are out and about in the country, in parks, or visiting other gardens and make a note of any details you find particularly pleasing, stimulating, inspiring or relaxing. Perhaps you may be able to create a similar area in your garden. In addition to an analysis of the bagua (see p. 18), it is a good idea to include some of these other factors in the plans for your garden. That way the garden will become a personal learning area where you can directly experience how your inner world and the outside world connect.

Reducing imbalance

Does your garden have buildings crowded on one side or does it have a large area of water on one side which creates a strong energetic charge? This will create an imbalance that may also lead to a one-sided extreme in the lives of the inhabitants. In order to balance this, you will need consciously to activate the weaker parts. Moving objects are particularly suitable for this, as movement means extra energy, like windmills, flags or plants whose leaves move in the slightest breeze. You can also use flowing water (see p. 34), lamps and gazing balls (see p. 36) or encourage wildlife into the garden (see p. 38).

Avoiding chi loss on slopes

If your garden is on a steep slope a downward dragging chi movement will occur. This drain can weaken the entire chi energy flow in the garden and create restlessness in your life. You should definitely try and stabilise this situation. Our ancestors tended to build terraces in these cases. The steps will hold and collect the chi, particularly if the edges of the terraces are equipped with plants. If terraces are out of the question, you should employ heavy garden elements on the slope like large boulders or stones, garden sculptures or plant troughs. This will help brake the chi flow and retain it in your garden. Features such as steps or a sloping terrace edges will prove invaluable.

The entrance to the garden

The entrance has a very special function as it not only provides access to all visitors but also determines the type of chi flow. It should be constructed to be suitably open and inviting. If possible, avoid placing a tree directly opposite the entrance as it will act as a barrier.

The garden path should be gently curving, built on firm foundations, and well lit (see p. 36). Planning the area in front

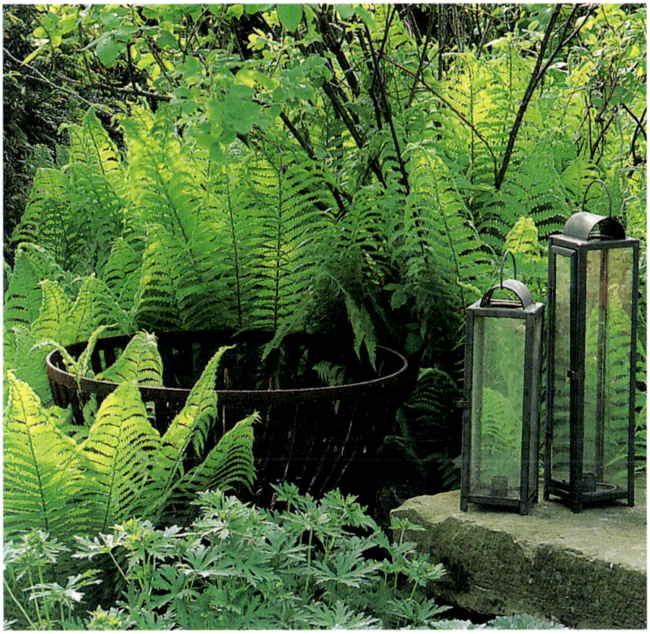

Light and shade – yin and yang.

of the house entrance in a circular or semi-circular design appears to have positive effects.

Retaining the chi

Fences, hedges or walls not only form boundaries around the plot but also keep the chi in the garden. They should not be made too massive, dense or tall, otherwise they will cut off the inhabitants from their surroundings. Wherever possible, do not introduce plants or structures that will hide beautiful views, and try to integrate the garden with its surroundings. Your life will also develop scope and open up in this way. Hedges with many types of wild plants and flowering plants are ideal for forming boundaries. Choose sloes (*Prunus spinosa*), apple rose (*Rosa rugosa*), dogwood (*Cornus mas*) and serviceberry (*Amelanchier laevis*), or evergreens like box (*Buxus sempervirens*, toxic) as well as common pyracantha (*Pyracantha coccinea*). These imaginative and attractive types of hedges will also provide food and shelter for wildlife.

A shady garden

There should be shady areas in the garden as well as sunny areas, according to the principles of yin and yang (see p. 10). Trees and bushes generally create plenty of shade under which the following will flourish: Bishop's hat (*Epimedium* species), *Saxifraga cortusifolia*, *Cimicifuga* species or decorative grasses like snowy woodrush (*Luzula nivea*). Terracotta containers will look good even in the shade if they are planted with geranium species, lady's mantle (*Alchemilla mollis*) or foam flower (*Tiarella cordifolia*).

Greenery on house walls

Allowing plants to grow over the walls of the house can positively influence the energy of the building. Windows and doors should not, however, be covered up. You should also choose a climbing plant you really like. This green coat will also balance temperature fluctuations and provide shelter for animals and insects. Popular species are ivy (*Hedera helix*, toxic), climbing roses (*Rosa* species), Boston ivy (*Parthenocissus tricuspidata*) or clematis species and hybrids.

A garden of the senses

Water is the main element of life. Without it plants, animals and humans would not be able to exist, as all life on Earth evolved from water.

It is also among the most important elements of a feng shui garden as it can collect energy and keep it flowing. The possibilities for design with water are endless. It enlivens the garden whether in the form of a pond, small stream, spring stone or a well. Specially designed catchment basins will even cause it to pulsate and raise the content of oxygen and energy.

Water also encourages wildlife to come into the garden – even a small birdbath will do – and you will get lot of pleasure from watching them.

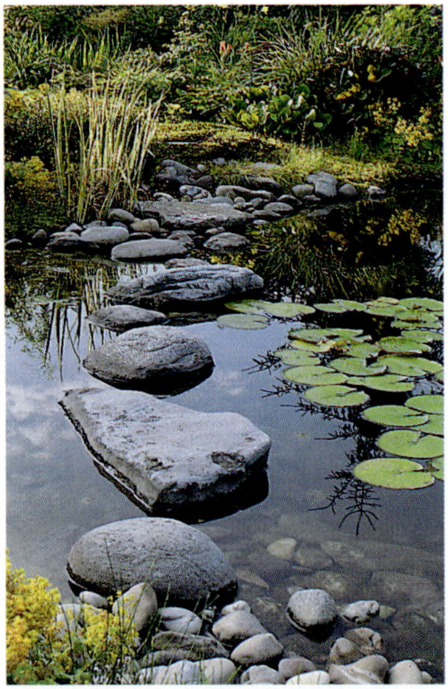

Stepping stones over a pond.

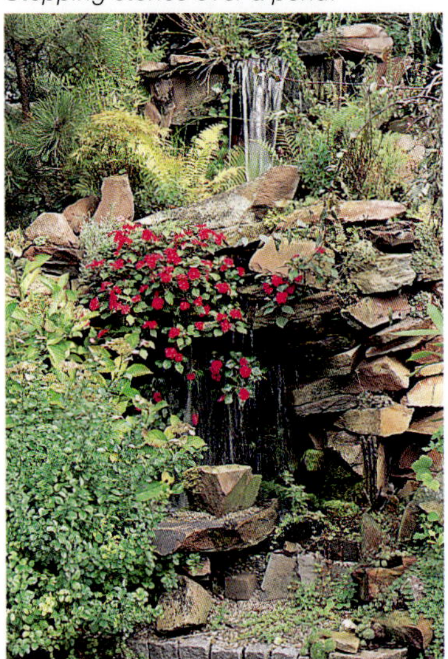

Miniature waterfall.

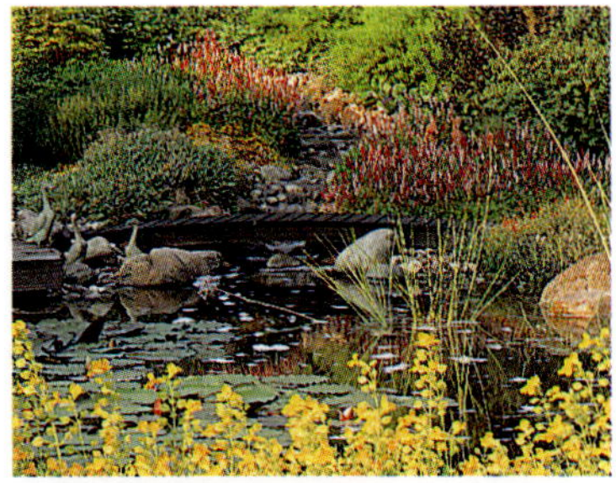

A simple wooden bridge.

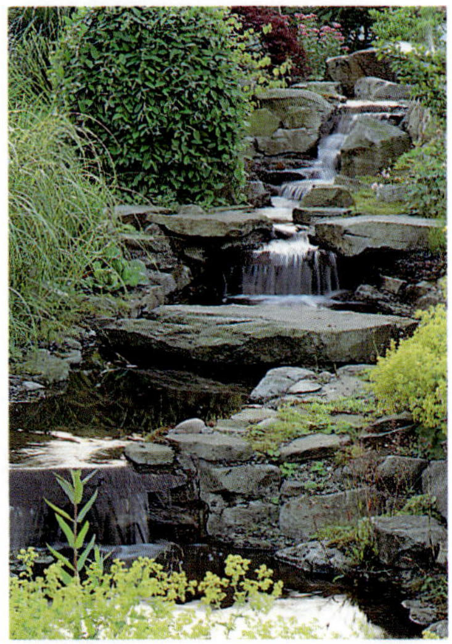

A stepped stream.

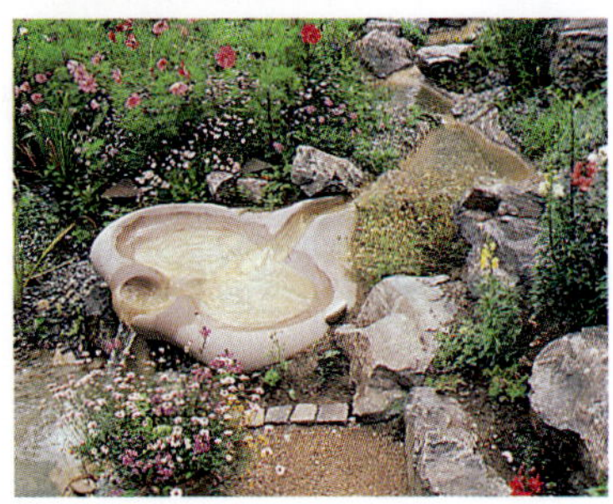

Catchment basins create soft ripples.

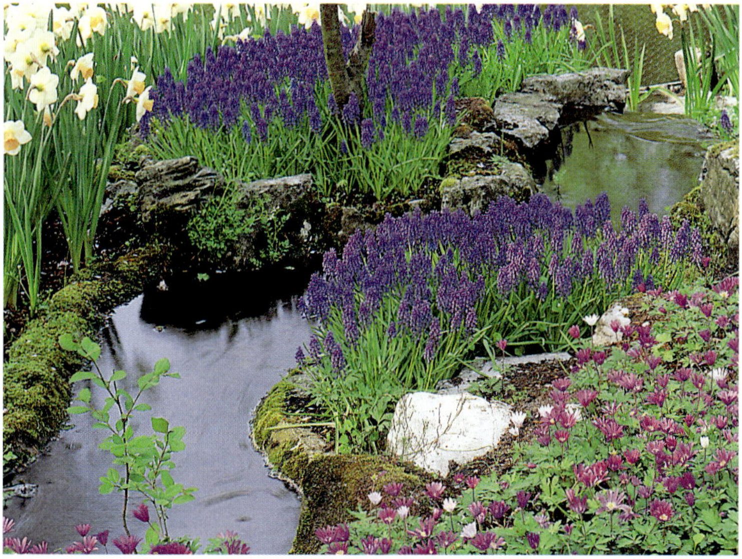

A gently curving stream, edged with flowers.

*The most important thing is for the water to be clean and clear. Make sure that it is not loaded with nutrients as this will cause algae to grow and the water will become muddy. Many plants like water crowfoot (*Ranunculus aquatilis*) will help keep the water clear. Running water contains a great deal of fresh oxygen and will not become muddy so easily.*

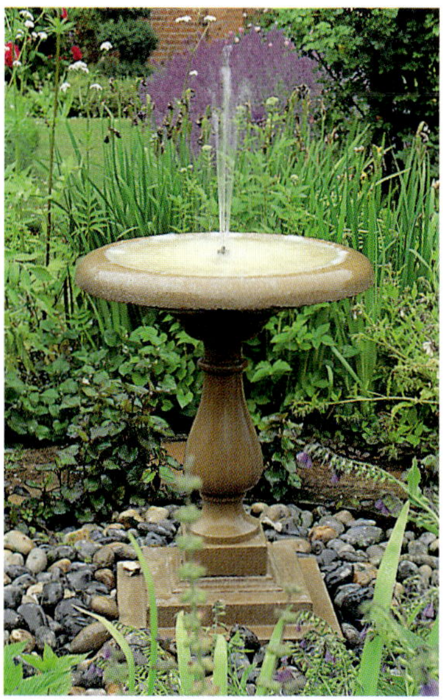

A sparkling fountain.

Allow yourself to be filled with the energy of fresh, clear water and enjoy its gentle splashing sound.

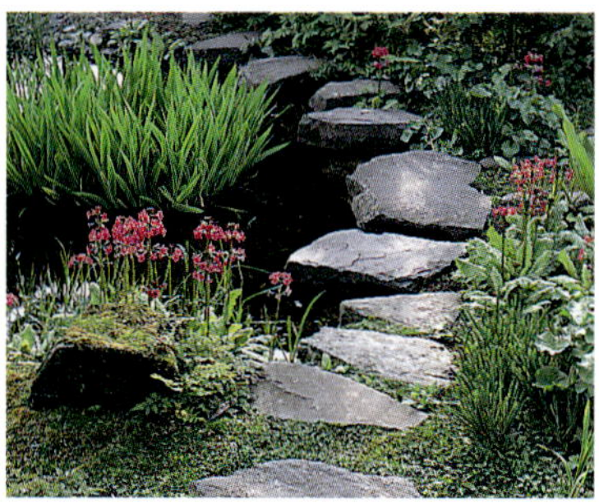

A path curves its way round a pond.

The magic of water

Water collects energy; flowing water in particular becomes charged with energy and will stimulate you. In the garden, there are many possibilities (see p. 32-33) to make use of it, preferably in the zones of Career, Family and Wealth (see p. 19):

- A pond of almost any size can be built; a natural pond sealed with clay would be ideal.
- A small man-made stream will make use of a natural or even an artificially built gradient and can be powered by installing a circulating pump.
- A waterfall can be created quite easily by installing an elevated step in the stream.
- Special catchment basins that are designed to create a pulsating, figure-of-eight wave motion can be obtained from special outlets. The shape of these basins creates an energy charge and the water movement is fascinating to watch.
- Spring stones or wells do not require a great deal of space and also release refreshing energy.
- Birdbaths made of stone or ceramic will fit into even the smallest garden. They also produce water energy and are inviting to many different species of birds.

Always make sure the quality of the water is good, as only healthy, clean water will increase the vibrations in your garden. Dirty water can have a negative effect on one's health or cause other adverse effects. A rule of thumb is that ponds with an area of more than six square metres that have been properly designed and equipped with plants will remain clean without care, whereas small installations that are driven with a circulating pump need regular checking and cleansing.

Important: In the case of water, the motto is too much is unhealthy. Do not install a large pond very close to the house as this very strong source of energy can be stressful in the long term.

Water veins and earth rays

Water veins and earth rays will also have a stressful effect on people in the long term. Living rooms should be completely free of them. You do not, however, normally spend all your time in the garden. If you have zones with good, clockwise energy in your garden, you may be able to establish your own personal energy spot there where you can tap into the intense energy for a quarter of an hour or so to fortify yourself. However, you should not sleep in this place.
How do you recognise an area where there are earth rays? Nature provides a few helpful hints: ants love to build their nests in places where these earth rays occur which is why, years ago, people used to release a sackful of ants on terrain where they wanted to build a shed, barn or farmhouse. If the ants disappeared quickly, it was all right to go ahead and build. Trees that are sensitive to radiation like apple, pear and cherry will often grow crooked or twisted in places with a lot of radiation. Radiation indicators or plants that seek such spots are, for example, ivy, elder, sea buckthorn and hazel. Box trees, and oaks are thought to alleviate the effects of radiation. They often grow in such places. You may wish to employ the services of an experienced dowser to check out the positions of earth currents and radiation on your site.

Labyrinths and spirals

Labyrinths and spirals have fascinated man for thousands of years. A distinction needs to be made between a labyrinth maze that has many cul-de-sacs and the classic labyrinth that has only one tortuous path running to the centre. The latter, just like the simple spiral, symbolises the eternal flow of life.
Both the labyrinth and the spiral generate a pulsating form of energy that moves inwards and outwards in waves.

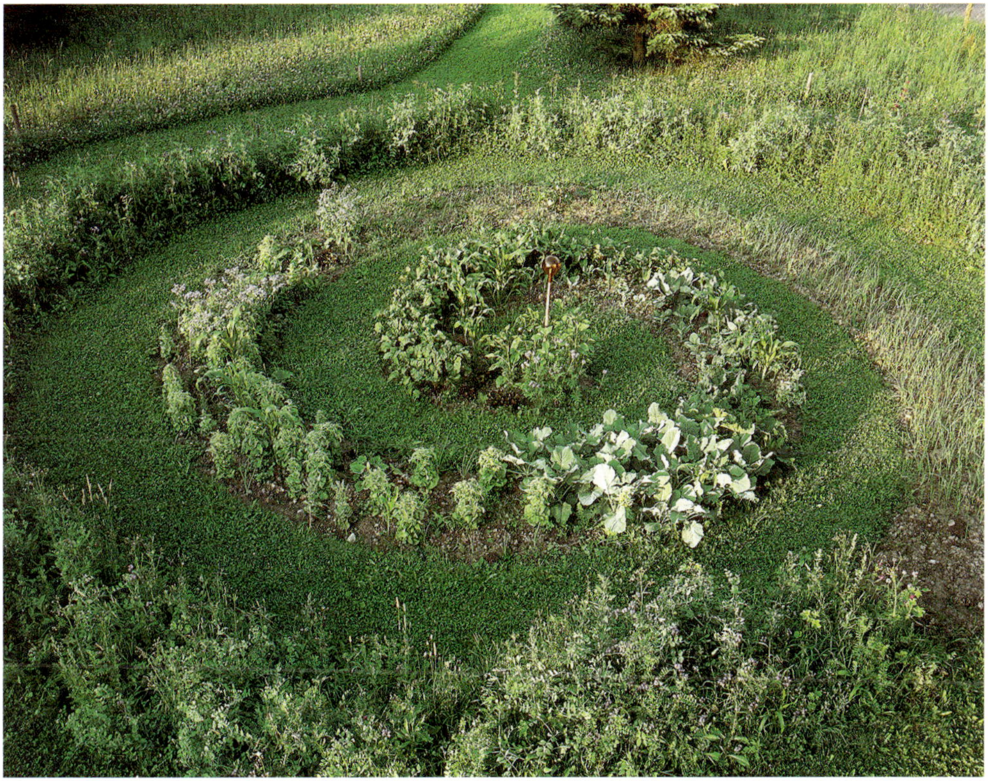

A spiral bed with mixed vegetables.

My Tip: If you wish to create this type of energy dispenser you should first make a sketch on paper and then transfer it, using sand or sawdust, onto the ground in the garden. This means you will still be able to make corrections quite easily before building it. There are many possibilities for designing if you want to combine flowers with lawn, vegetables with soil, or box trees with gravel or coloured sand. There is more information about herb spirals on p. 42-43.

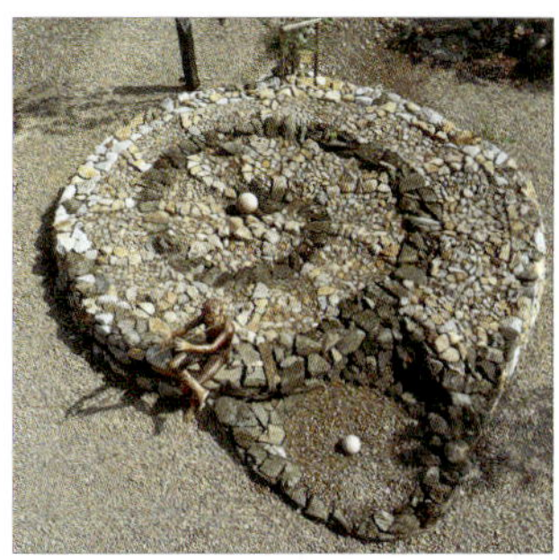

A spiral rockery.

Paths – chi veins

Paths are energy-conducting connecting veins between the different parts of the garden. They should always be gently curving, wide enough and built on firm foundations, in order to allow a free energy flow. Straight paths would accelerate the chi too much (see p. 10). But also make sure that no inhibiting branches jut out over the path. Soft, natural-looking groups of plants along the edges of paths are also recommended.

My Tip: In the case of wide, straight paths, you can allow plants to grow out onto the surface of the path at intervals on alternate sides or place plants in round containers at intervals along the edges in order to achieve a more curving course.

Directions of paths. Skillfully designed connecting paths will also create a sense of distance in even the smallest areas, shielding your garden from any threatening energies from its surroundings. Paths that lead to a quiet area or a peaceful marginal area of the garden, can be a little simpler and narrower without causing detriment.

Important: In the case of strong and possibly disturbing influences from outside you should avoid any kind of direct connection of paths (see p. 24).

Materials. Use predominantly natural materials for the surfacing and make sure it is safe to walk on. Choose colours that encourage the mood or atmosphere you desire.
Steps. They should be built securely and be well lit from dusk onwards. The chi flow can be accelerated where the gradient is high. We recommend placing heavy, braking objects like containers with plants or large rocks or boulders on the half-landings along steps (see p. 30).
Bridges. These gather the chi together, conduct it across ditches or water, and have a connecting, stabilising effect. They also add a special magical touch to your garden.

Covered walks

If you make a leafy tunnel or an arch over a path, you will create a strong zone of vitality. Walking underneath a rose arch or spending the afternoon in the cool shade of an arbour has a healing effect on the mind, soul and body. In open gardens that one can look into from the outside, an arbour covered with climbing plants and leafy creepers provides a visual screen and intimacy. Various different areas of the garden (see p. 25) can be improved with covered walks.
Suitable climbing plants are woody plants like climbing roses (*Rosa*), clematis hybrids, honeysuckle (*Lonicera caprifolium*), *Polygonum aubertii* and *Parthenocissus quinquefolia* as well as annuals like scented sweet pea (*Lathyrus odoratus*), runner beans (*Phaseolus coccineus*) and black-eyed Susans (*Thunbergia alata*).

Lighting in the garden

Atmospheric lighting along curving paths should enable one to use the garden safely even in the dark. Naturally, the same goes for the house entrance where you will use light as a kind of link to the outside world. More energy can be brought into the garden areas of Fame, Partnership, Knowledge and the Centre (see p. 21) by means of lighting. It is fine to switch the lights on just when you need them, but ideally, there could be a timer which automatically switches on the lights at dusk. A light can also have a balancing effect if a bagua zone is missing entirely (see p. 48).

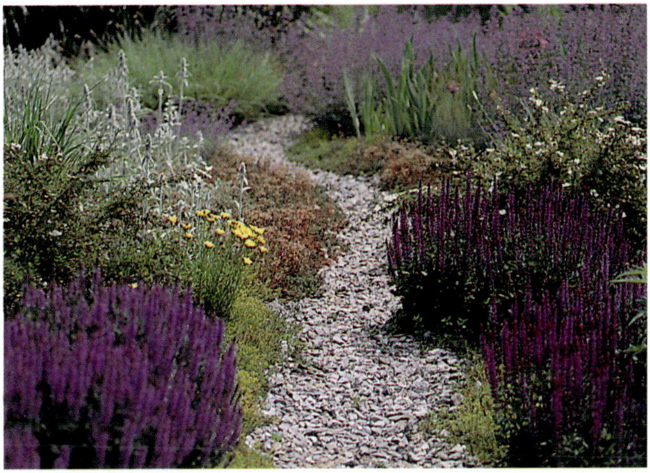
Flowering plants frame this winding gravel path.

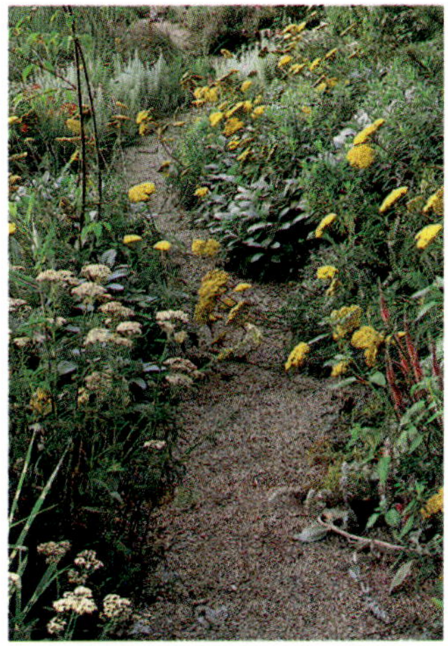
Sandy path.

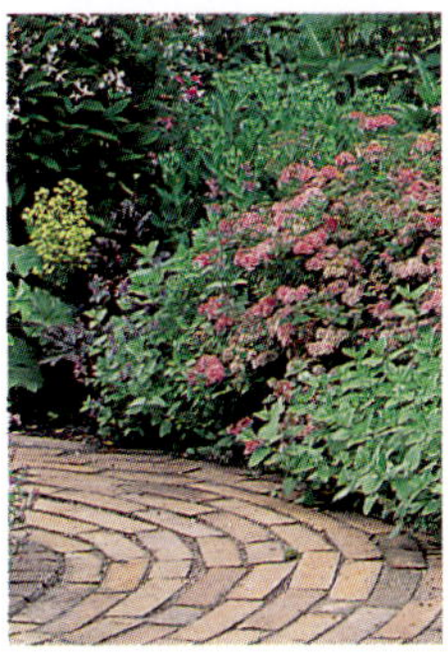
Curving brick path.

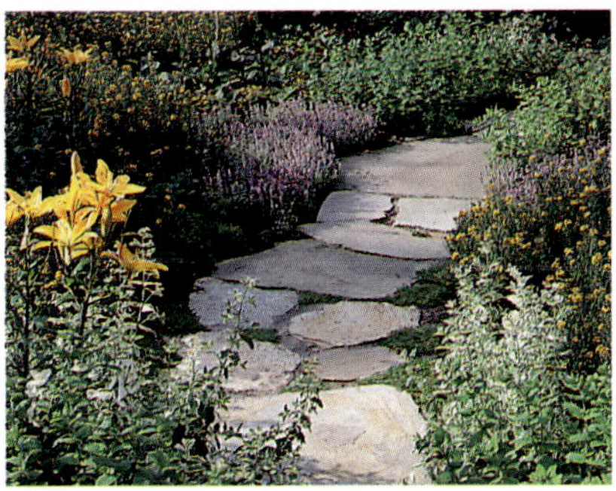
Natural flagstones: sturdy and solid.

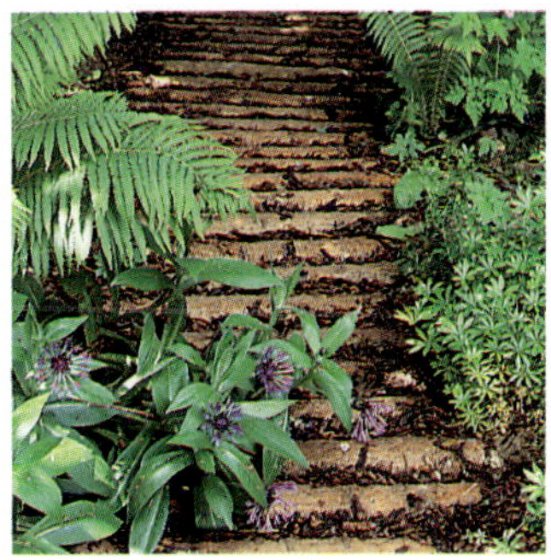
Wooden decking.

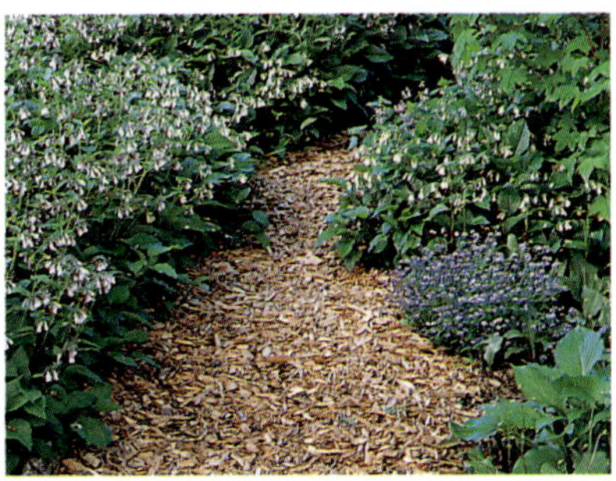
Path covered in bark chips.

Harmonious paths

If your paths run in gentle curves and are not blocked by anything they will act like veins, allowing nourishing energy to flow through the garden. Build them from natural, local materials if possible.

Enjoying with all five senses

The perfect feng shui garden is also a garden of the senses, designed to be an antidote to the diminishing opportunities for sensual perception in everyday life. Such a garden will open up and awaken your consciousness to new aspects of life and even memories that disappeared years ago, start to be awakened once again.
None of the senses is meant to predominate, as all five senses play such a fundamental part in our communication with the outside world. They are all equally important – even if we tend to attribute more importance to our eyesight than anything else. In a feng shui garden all five senses should be addressed and you will find more on this in the following pages.

Seeing

If you choose the shapes and

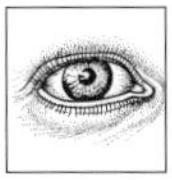

colours of plants according to the principles of yin and yang (see p. 10) and the elements (see p. 21), you will discover new visual attractions wherever you tread in your garden. Different heights of growth and varying denser or more open planting, as well as contrasts between pale and dark colours, light and shade, have a refreshing effect on the eye. Colourful flowers appear particularly conspicuous if they are surrounded by areas of calm shades of green. Inspiration is also encouraged if you allow the eye to gain in-depth views with curving pathways and staggered arrangements of plants. Also, design the seating area in the garden in such a way that the gaze falls comfortably on particularly beautiful details like a bizarre shaped stone, running water or or a particularly decorative woody area.
When planning the garden, take account of the seasonal change of colours, and combine the deciduous species with evergreen species so that the view from the window will include splashes of colour in the garden even in winter.
Cut flowers. Do not forget plants that can be grown for cut flowers when choosing plants. They are like a fresh gift from the garden and will fill your living area or the garden table with colour. You will derive far more pleasure from flowers you have grown in your garden than from bought bouquets.

Watching animals

Watching animals and birds make themselves at home in your garden will give you a lot of pleasure. You can be sure that good chi is present wherever animals feel comfortable. For this reason, it is a good idea to create ideal conditions for birds by hanging up nesting boxes or creating nesting possibilities in hedges and planting trees like mountain ash *(Sorbus aucuparia)* so the birds can feed on its berries. Secluded areas of the garden that are left in their natural state are ideal habitats for small mammals like hedgehogs and other creatures like lizards and insects.
Rockeries and dry-stone walls also give good shelter for all kinds of wildlife.

My tip: Those parts of the garden that are activated with running water, a fountain, for example, during the warm part of the year, can be be equipped with a substitute source of energy in the winter by attracting birds. Areas of the garden where seeds and grain are put out for the birds are considered to be particularly activated. You will also be able to activate a lot of chi in this way in a newly designed garden.

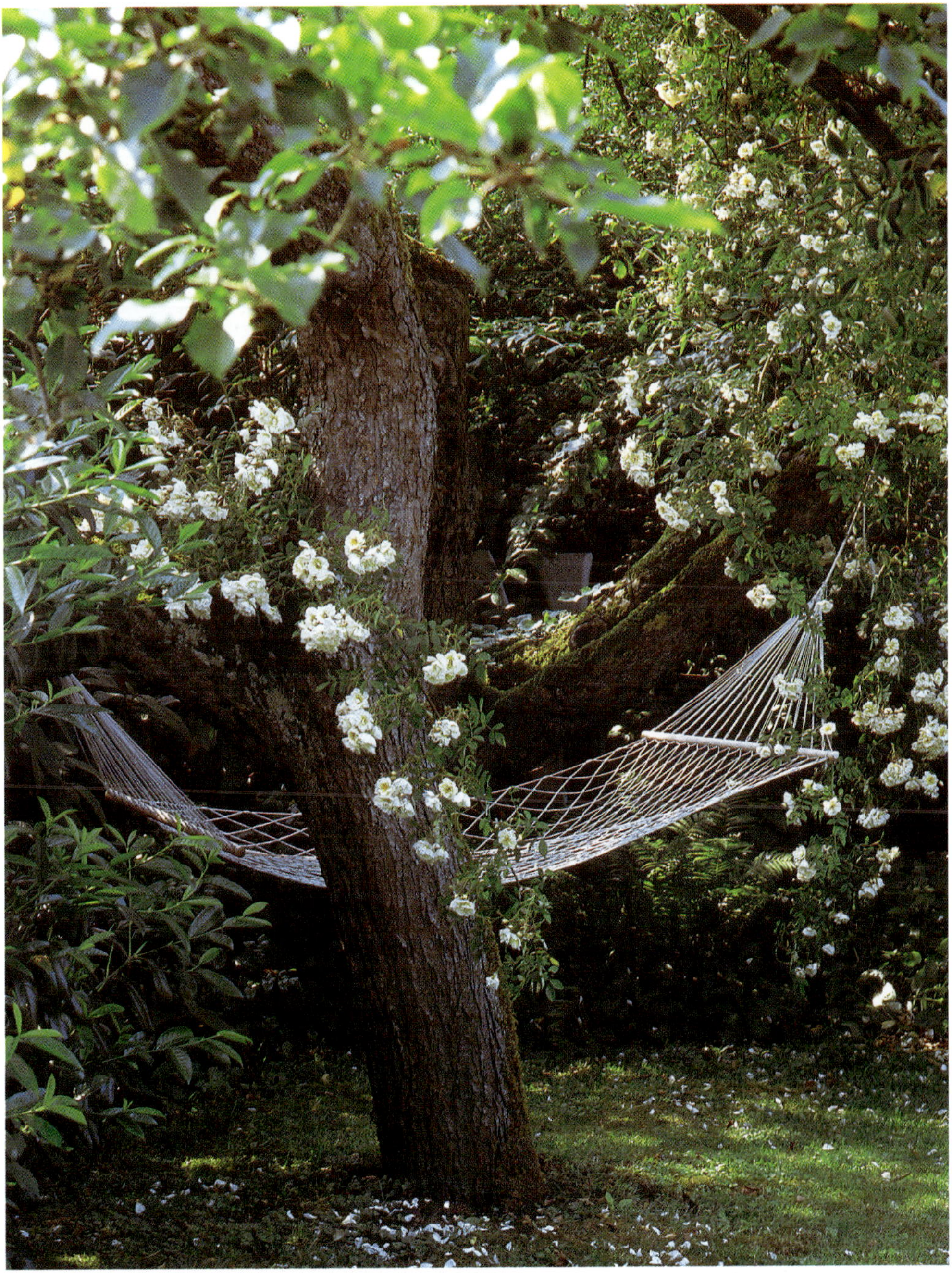

Relax in a hammock and enjoy your surroundings with all your senses.

A garden of the senses

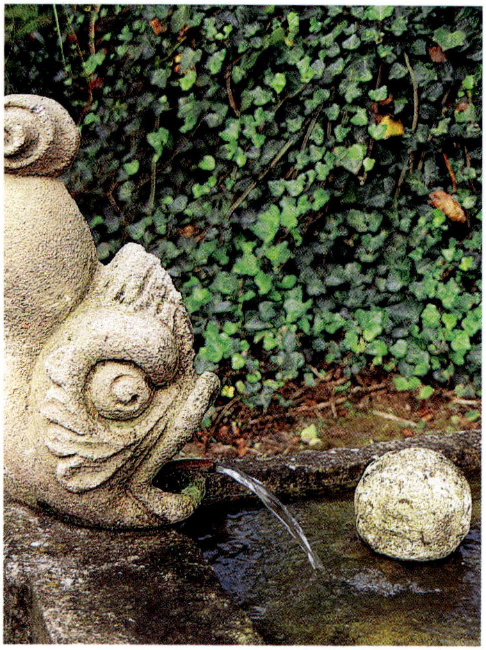

A calming trickle of water.

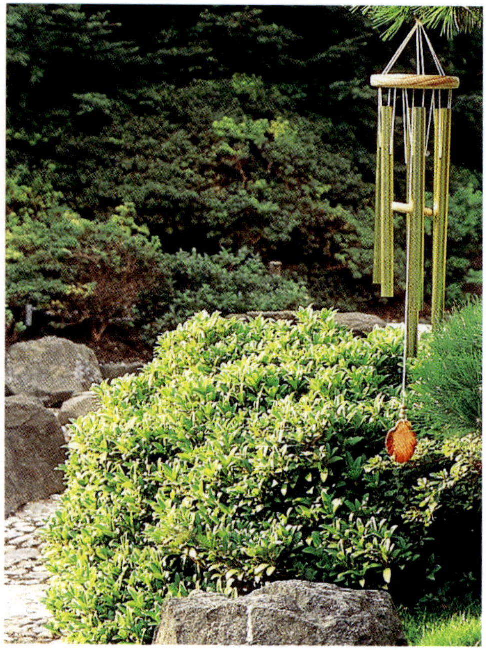

Wind chimes with harmonising notes.

Hearing

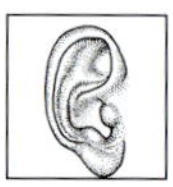

Increasing noise pollution from our environment is having a dramatically detrimental effect on our potential for hearing things, as it decreases the facility for perceiving high and low frequencies. The result is that your voice also reduces its range of sounds and only those frequencies that the ear can hear are able to be expressed with the human voice. This, in turn, reduces our facility for communicating and we end up living at a 'low frequency'. You will be able to work against this fatal cycle by training your ears and transforming your garden into a paradise of sound. The rustling of leaves in the wind, the gentle trickle of a waterfall, the murmuring of a stream at the edge of a path, the splashing of a spring stone beside a sitting place, the paddling sound of a waterwheel installed especially for the children, the twittering of birds for whom you have created a good habitat, or even the quiet chirping of grasshoppers in the heat of a summer's evening will consciously encourage your sense of hearing again.

Wind chimes

Gentle chiming not only has a relaxing effect but also inspires and activates the immune system. Birch (*Betula* species) and bamboo (*Phyllostachys* species) with the light silvery sounds of their constantly moving leaves act like natural wind chimes.
They create a particularly light,

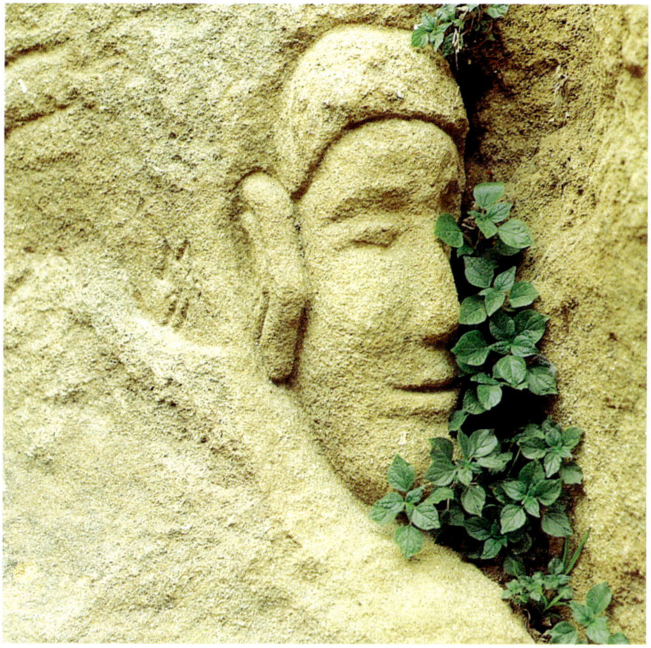

Rough, hewn stone – good for touching and feeling.

airy vibration. Even a bought set of wind chimes made of metal pipes, wood, bamboo cane, shells or ceramic hung up in your favourite tree, will create atmospheric and therapeutic sounds. Chimes that spread a wave-shaped vibration are assigned to the element Water (see p. 21) and are, therefore, particularly suitable for energising the areas of Career, Wealth and Family.

Touching

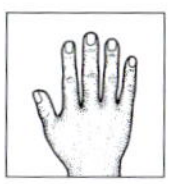

Our sense of touch has also been greatly reduced in our, 'smooth', modern environment. Even basic sensory needs like body contact and stroking are increasingly substituted by other actions, whether through the handling of soft toys, fabric softeners in a washing machine or visits to the hairdresser, beautician or masseur. Learn how to grasp your life more intensely by creating an area in your garden for touching, feeling and stroking. A place like this will also strengthen the chi of visitors. Polished, rough or hewn stones, textured wood surfaces, wavy handrails, materials that warm up and cool down at different rates, stiff and flexible plants, rough or smooth plants, rough or glossy leaves, sand that you can run through your fingers or with which your children can make sand pies, sea shells and snail shells, chestnuts and cones for fingering, walking barefoot in the garden, walking through morning dew or over a gravel path...the possibilities are endless in a garden.

My tip: Touching makes you more touchable. You will be astonished at how much more intensely you will feel the world about you. Your garden will become even more attractive and your experience of your surroundings will become even more intense through the additional possibilities of sensual perception and experience. The result will be lots of positive chi.

A garden of the senses

A sense of smell

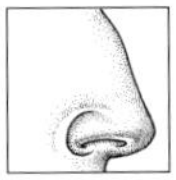

Synthetically manufactured scented substances now dominate our everyday lives. Smells influence us on a very subtle level. In the USA, clever estate agents actually try and influence potential buyers with the help of scented sprays squirted in houses to make them smell cosy and motivate the customer to come to a faster decision. It is obvious that this flood of sensory input must happen at the cost of our finer ability to smell and increasingly people complain that there are many things they cannot smell anymore or that things 'get up their noses'. Fresh, natural scents create a balance here. Depending on the plant, they can have a stimulating, calming, aphrodisiacal or refreshing effect or may stimulate the body's natural immune systems. The right scent can be found for practically all needs. Try to create a temple of scents in your garden – even if it is very small. Buy with your nose and choose herbs, flowers and bushes according to their scent. Create your own personal pot pourri; depending on the time of day – morning and evening smells are very different – and the time of year, you will be able to enjoy a whole range of scents in your garden.

Herbs

Herbs and healing plants should be present in every feng shui garden. They spread a kind of aromatic magic about them and actually stimulate neighbouring plants to an increased production of scents. The ideal position for a herb collection is the south as it will then positively influence the entire garden and its inhabitants. It can, however, work well in any other position in the garden.

Herb spiral. A spiral herb garden is built like a dry-stone wall out of natural stone in a spiral shape, rising up gradually, and offers different living habitats in a very small space in which a colourful mixture of herbs will flourish particularly well. It is not only an attractive feature, its shape will also ensure that the power field around the plants is increased. The lower part of the spiral is good for moisture-loving herbs like lemon balm (*Melissa officinalis*), peppermint (*Mentha* x *piperita*) and *Nasturtium officinale*. In the middle section we find marjoram (*Origanum majorana*), basil (*Ocimum basilicum*), chives (*Allium schoenoprasum*), hyssop (*Hyssopus officinalis*) and parsley (*Petroselinum crispum*). In the upper levels, finally, we come across the plants that love dryness and sunlight, like sage (*Salvia officinalis*), thyme (*Thymus vulgaris*), savory (*Satureja montana*) and rosemary (*Rosmarinus officinalis*). If you would like to know more about herb spirals and how to build them, you will find more detailed information in the herb book recommended on p. 62.

Scented plants

Scented species can be found outside the kingdom of herbs, especially among flowering plants. Among them are annuals like scented sweet pea (*Lathyrus odoratus*) or *Reseda odorata* and perennials like lavender (*Lavandula angustifolia*), sweet rocket (*Hesperis matronalis*), catmint (*Nepeta x faassenii*) or *Dianthus plumarius*. Even among the woody plants one will find many scented ones like roses (*Rosa* species), lilac (*Syringa vulgaris*) or scented snowball (*Viburnum fragrans*).

Then there are a few decorative plants of which the leaves in particular have a strong fragrance, for instance, cotton lavender (*Santolina chamaecyparissus*) and *Monarda* hybrids. Many of these plants do not release a proper scent until you stroke them with your hand or rub the leaves. The best place for them is along the edges of paths where the scent is released when you pass. It is easier to appreciate scented flowers if you grow them in

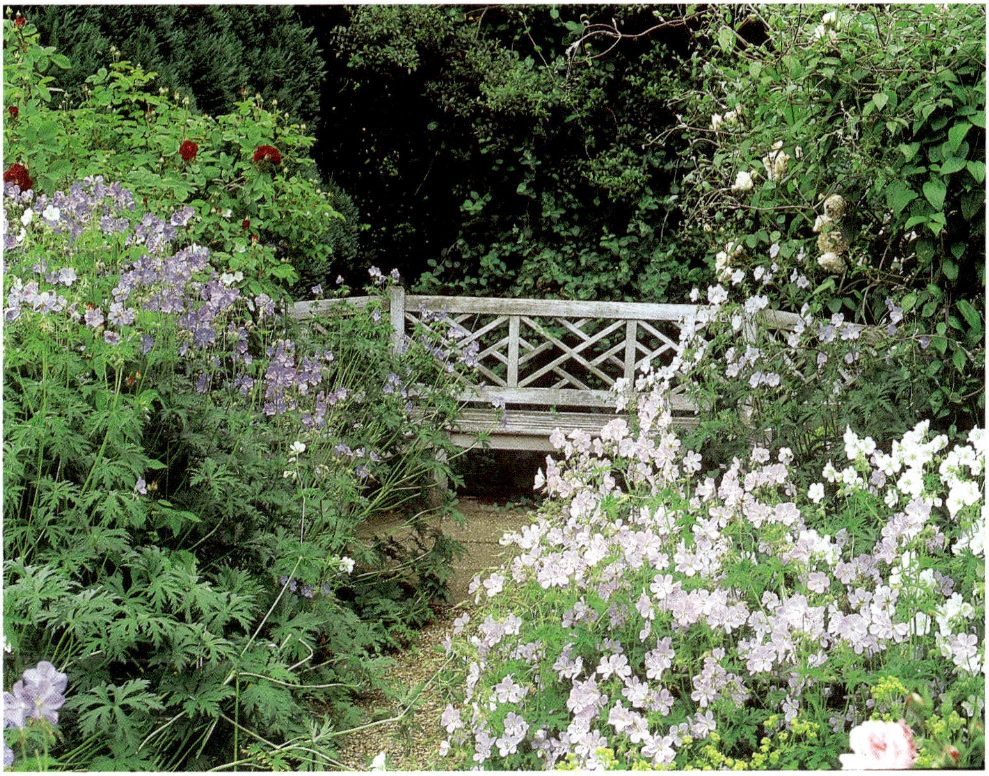

The perfect place to sit, surrounded by sweet-smelling flowers.

raised beds where you can reach to smell the petals. Try to include plenty of scented plants near your sitting corner.

Important: Do not place strong-smelling plants directly under the window of a bedroom or study as sensitive people are prone to get headaches from the strong scents.

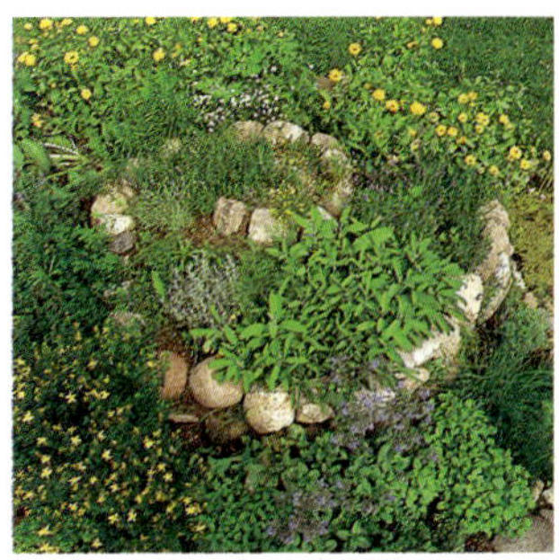

Herb spirals generate energy.

Tasting

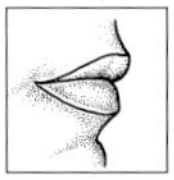

The garden can offer an enormous range of taste experiences, the huge potential of which is still not fully realised. Herbs, vegetables and berry bushes can be well integrated even in a small decorative garden. They taste a lot stronger if they are freshly harvested and they contain more vitamins and minerals than bought groceries. The chi is also incomparably better. If you follow the growth of the plants until the harvest and have been looking forward to enjoying them long before they are ripe, your immediate sense of taste will also be heightened. Home-grown food is enjoyed with quite a different kind of consciousness, the taste becomes far more important. Herbs from your own garden also increase the sense of taste.

Enjoy caring for the garden

You will enjoy your garden much more, and it will be much easier to maintain if you place the plants in suitable positions and care for them in harmony with nature. Here are the most important considerations for a low-maintenance garden.

Mixed culture

This is a natural growing method in which vegetables, in particular, encourage each other and protect each other from pests and can be grown in a space-saving community of plants. Carrots *(Daucus carota)* and onions (*Allium cepa)* will flourish in this way and will help each other ward off the carrot fly and the onion fly. Then there is leek *(Allium porrum)* and lettuce *(Lactuca sativa)*. Some plants harmonise less well, like carrots and celery *(Apium graveolens)* or leeks and beans *(Phaseolus vulgaris)*. Most good books on vegetable cultivation will include tables to show favourable and unfavourable vegetable combinations.

Composting

Compost is also extremely important in feng shui teaching. To ensure optimal maturing it should be mixed well and regularly forked over. Adding bonemeal encourages the breakdown of the organic matter. Elder (*Sambucus nigra)* is particularly suited to providing shade and will pass its healing vibrations on to the compost. Elder can also cope with a good dollop of compost while fruit trees will often not bear much fruit in this position because they will receive too many nutrients. It is also a good idea to allow a few stinging nettles *(Urtica dioica)* to grow beside the compost heap, they help control aphids and are also a versatile healing plant.

Slugs and snails

Whenever a pest becomes particularly conspicuous it is usually a sign of an imbalance in nature. Slugs and snails will only really attack plants whose life energy is weakened. This is not only the case with sick plants but also with freshly planted young plants or seedlings. Protect them with a ring of dry sawdust, set up beer traps or lay shoots of yarrow, tansy or tomatoes around, as slugs and snails hate the smell of all these plants. Experience has also shown that slugs and snails cause far less damage in spiral shaped vegetable beds.

Fortifying plants naturally

Whenever pests start appearing, you should use organic plant extracts instead of chemical substances.

- Nettles, fern or wormwood are helpful in controlling aphids.
- Spraying with a non-toxic soft soap solution is also very effective.

Depending on the degree of infestation, dissolve 150 to 300 g pure soft soap from the chemists in 10 litres hot water. After it has cooled down leave it undiluted and spray the infested plants.

- Tansy or tomatoes are good against caterpillar infestation.
- Tansy or dusting with bonemeal are helpful against flea beetles.
- Both tansy and wormwood

(*Artemesia*) will get rid of spider mites.

● Mare's tail is effective against mildew and rust.

Further instructions and information can be found in organic gardening books.

Care in the autumn

The highly active potential of the garden in the spring and summer gradually decreases towards the autumn when nature is preparing for its winter rest. Annual plants will die down completely, but generally produce seed. In the case of perennials, the parts above ground will generally die back but underground, in the roots, bulbs or tubers, life will survive. Among the woody species, the evergreen ones will now dominate beside the bare but still living branches and twigs of the deciduous species. For the sake of the wildlife, do not clear up too efficiently in the autumn. During winter you will not spend so much time in your garden and will tend to admire it more from your windows. Do not start composting dead parts of plants until the spring.

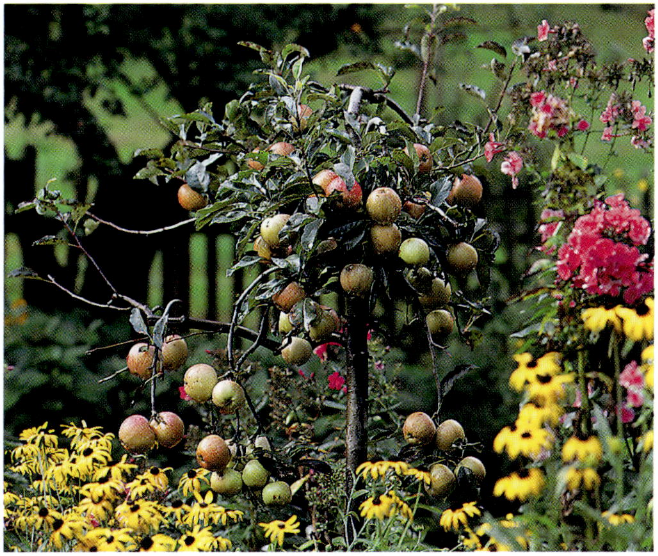

Deliciously ripe apples, fresh from the garden.

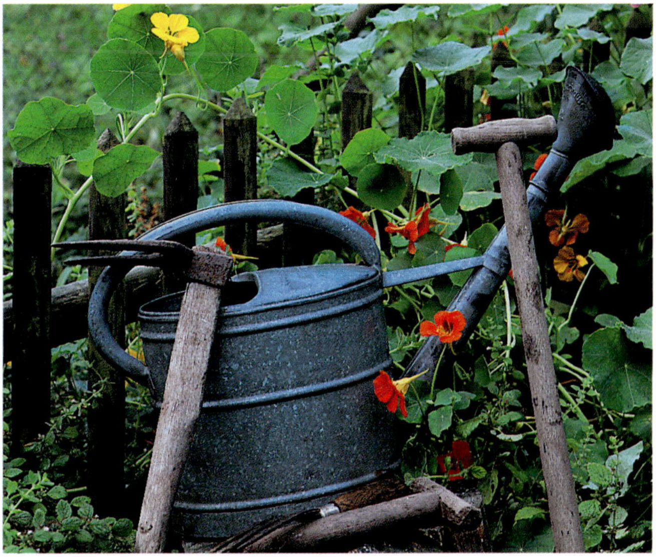

Caring for your garden can be very rewarding.

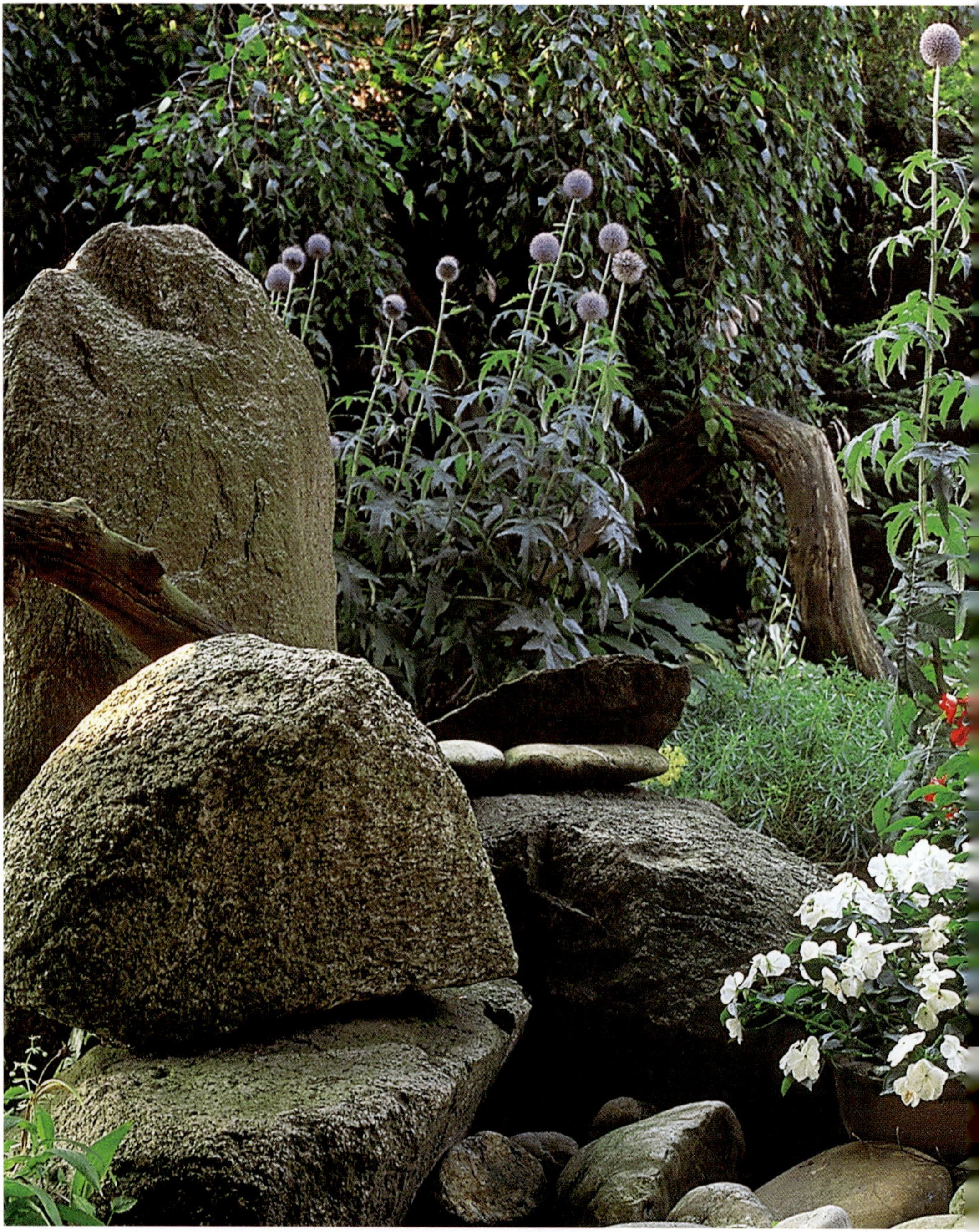

Enhancing the bagua zones

Making changes

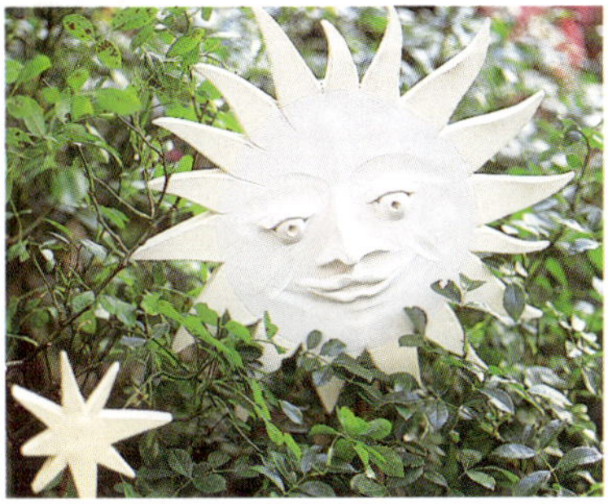

This sun shines in all weathers.

You may have found out, with the help of the bagua and by looking closely at your own life, that one zone or even several areas in your garden need improving. This chapter explains how to redesign and improve these areas and how you can balance their weaknesses.

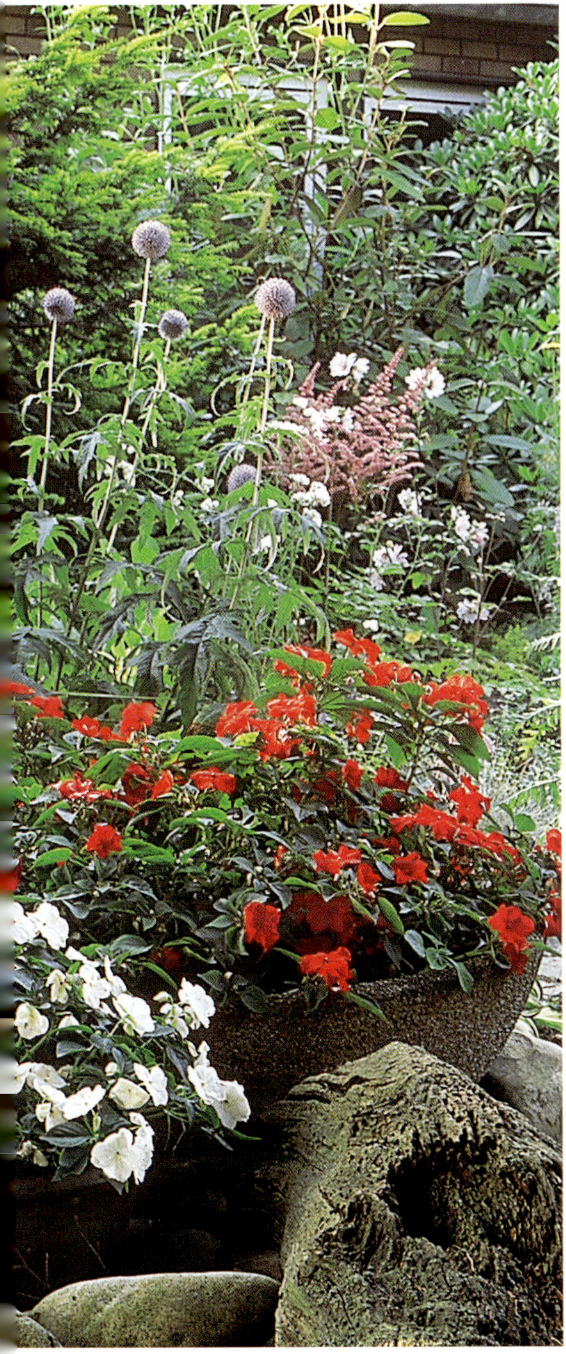

A place of power – with natural rocks and plenty of flowering plants.

What changes should be made?

Try looking at your garden from different angles and you will soon realise what needs to be done:

- Look for the four heavenly animals in your garden (see p. 11).
- Lay the bagua sheet on a ground plan of your garden and then determine where the individual zones are (see p. 16-19).
- Analyse the area surrounding your garden with the help of the questionnaires on p. 24-25.
- Gain clarity about your own inner condition with the help of the questionnaires on p. 26-27.
- Do not forget to listen to your own inner voice: take a quiet walk around your garden, look at the land and the plants and listen inwardly. What appeals to you, speaks to you, what fills you with restlessness, is there anything you dislike?

Changes will always be necessary if:

- The four heavenly animals are not properly defined (see p. 12).
- You discover, after studying the table on p. 21 (remedy, see p. 22), that inhibiting influences are present in one or several bagua zones.
- The questionnaire on p. 24-25 shows that damaging influences from the surroundings or from the garden itself need to be dealt with.
- The questionnaire on p. 26-27 indicates that the flow of your life could do with some changes.
- Your inner voice tells you that changes are needed.

Weak or missing bagua zones

In the case of very irregularly shaped gardens, one or several bagua zones may be only minimally or partly present. This amounts to a weakness or total lack (see p. 18).
Weak zones can be fortified by intensively employing the elements assigned to that zone (see p. 21) in the form of colours, accessories or plants.
Missing areas can be improved by placing a lamp on the boundary of the property so that the light acts as a balancing feature. In this case, it will connect your garden with the bagua zone that is situated on your neighbour's plot. It will be sufficient to allow the lamp to burn for a few hours in the evening. Gazing balls made of coloured glass have a very similar effect. Their entire surroundings are mirrored in their surfaces and the curved surface reflects away again.
My tip: Gazing balls are generally well suited, due to the properties described, to draw nourishing chi out of the surroundings and to protect the plot from stressful influences in the surroundings. The globes have a particularly strong effect if they are employed in pairs, for example, left and right of the path, by a fence or beside a garden gate.

Splendid colours

Do you have a little space to spare in the bagua zone you want to strengthen? You could employ accessories and plants in the colours that belong both to the element assigned to this zone as well as to the supportive element (see p. 21). In the case of Wood and Water, for example, these would be delicate graded shades of light to medium to blackish blue, in the case of Fire and Wood, they would be rich contrasts of red and green to medium blue. In the case of Water and Metal, use noble pairings of black, dark blue, white, silver and gold, and for Earth and Fire, employ a lively combination of yellow, orange and red. The following pages include more information about the many different design possibilities for the individual bagua zones and also about recommended alterations.

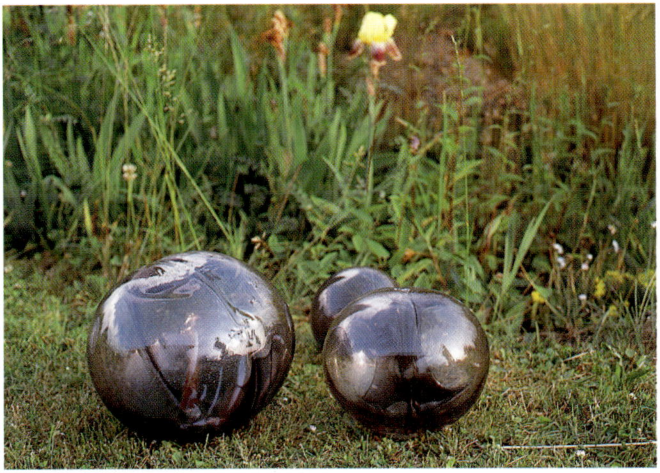

Gazing balls, this time on a lawn.

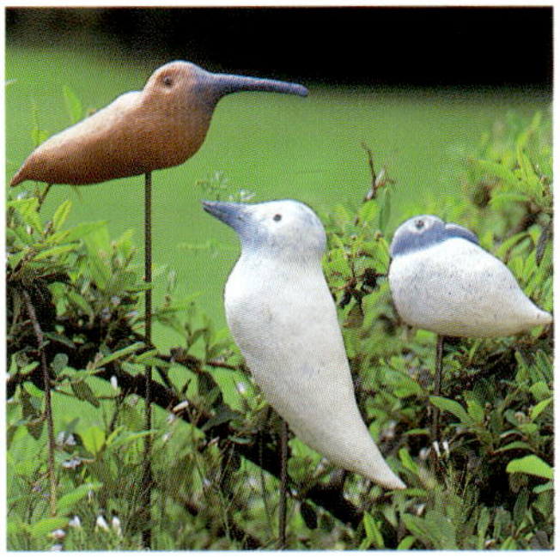

Ceramic birds.

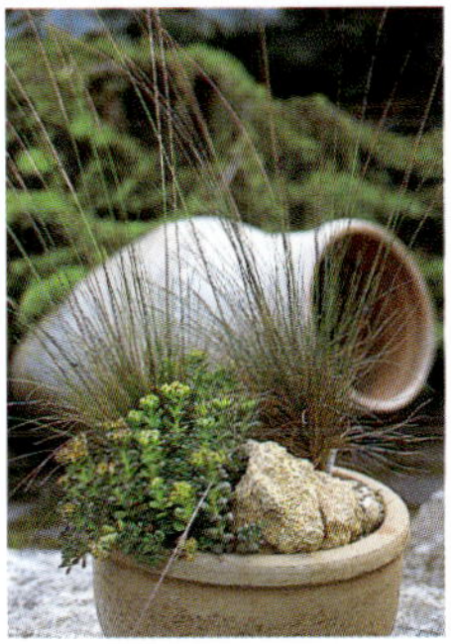

Terracotta containers.

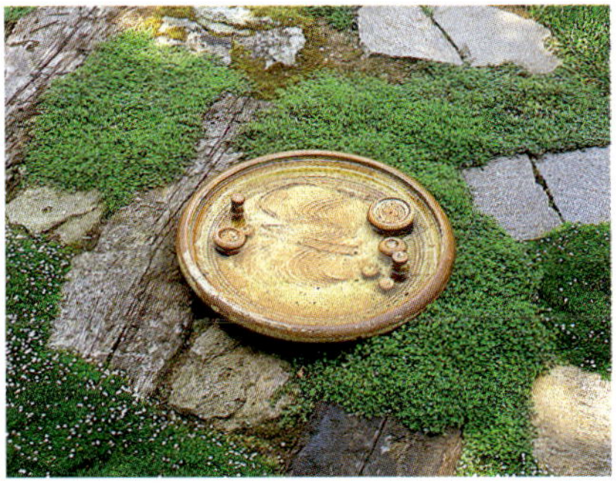

Ceramic birdbath.

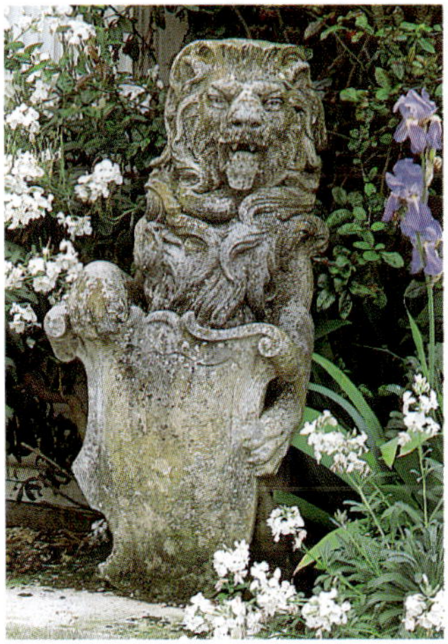

A stone lion.

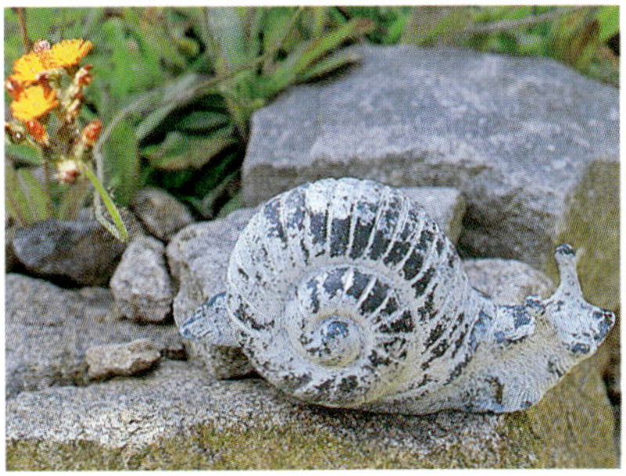

Decorative metal snail.

Accessories to enhance energy flow

There are so many attractive garden accessories to be found and they need not be expensive. Even one single addition, well chosen, may radically alter the energy flow in your garden and will often make further alterations unnecessary.

Knowledge

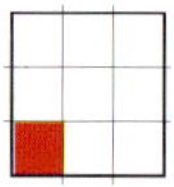

This zone lies to the outer left of the base line of the bagua. It is assigned to the element Earth with the colours yellow, orange, brown (see p. 21). The element Fire has an encouraging effect with the colours pink, red or wine red, while Wood has an inhibiting effect with the colours green and light to medium blue. If you were planning to design a children's play area in this zone, it could lead to turbulence in your life as this particular area of the garden should radiate a great deal of peace. Ensure that there are lots of plants growing here – which is often in the front garden – and that they are specially dense and visually impenetrable. Avoid using too many column-shaped plants that are assigned to the inhibiting element Wood. Plant low-growing, ground cover plants, such as broom (*Genista lydia*) and alyssum *(Alyssum saxatile*). If possible, leave space for a hidden, cave-like seating place between the trees and bushes at a safe distance from sources of noise. Make yourself a quiet contemplative spot, screened from the curious eyes of passers-by and away from other disturbances. You will be amazed at its beneficial effect. Hollow stones and other objects with hollows are also valuable feng shui devices for the Knowledge zone. Even a small tool shed would be well placed in this zone.

Career

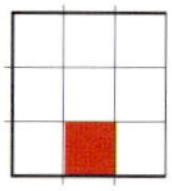

This zone lies at the centre of the base line of the bagua, often near the entrance. It is assigned to the element Water with the colours dark blue to black. The supportive element is Metal with the colours white, silver and gold, while the element Earth with the colours yellow, orange and brown has an inhibiting effect.

The chi should be able to move easily in the zone as it represents your life flow. Curved beds are suitable, a lightly wavy shape of terrain and plants that give the same impression. Running water is also good here or if there is not much space, a spring stone could be designed. Where there is more room, install a small stream, or perhaps even special catchment basins (see p. 34). Try to reduce the number of accessories that are assigned to the inhibiting element Earth (see table on p. 23).

Helpful people

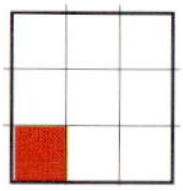

This zone is situated on the right of the base line. It is assigned to the element Metal with the colours white, silver and gold. The element Earth has an enhancing effect with the colours yellow, orange, brown, and the element Fire is inhibiting together with the colours pink, red and wine red. This zone symbolises the active and intense exchange with the surroundings. It is a good place for a cosy sitting area to share with friends. This garden area can be activated successfully with beautiful stones or garden lamps. Avoid using too much of the inhibiting element Fire.

Where to put your car? One possible place is the Helpful people zone. Any vehicle will have a tendency to create a disturbing influence on the garden. Make sure that parking spaces are hidden with a visual screen of plants, which will also help to restore balance. You can also screen the dustbins here. A wooden car port is preferable to a garage and you could train climbing plants over it. Do not design the drive to be too straight and, if possible, avoid concrete or asphalt surfaces – use grass grid blocks instead.

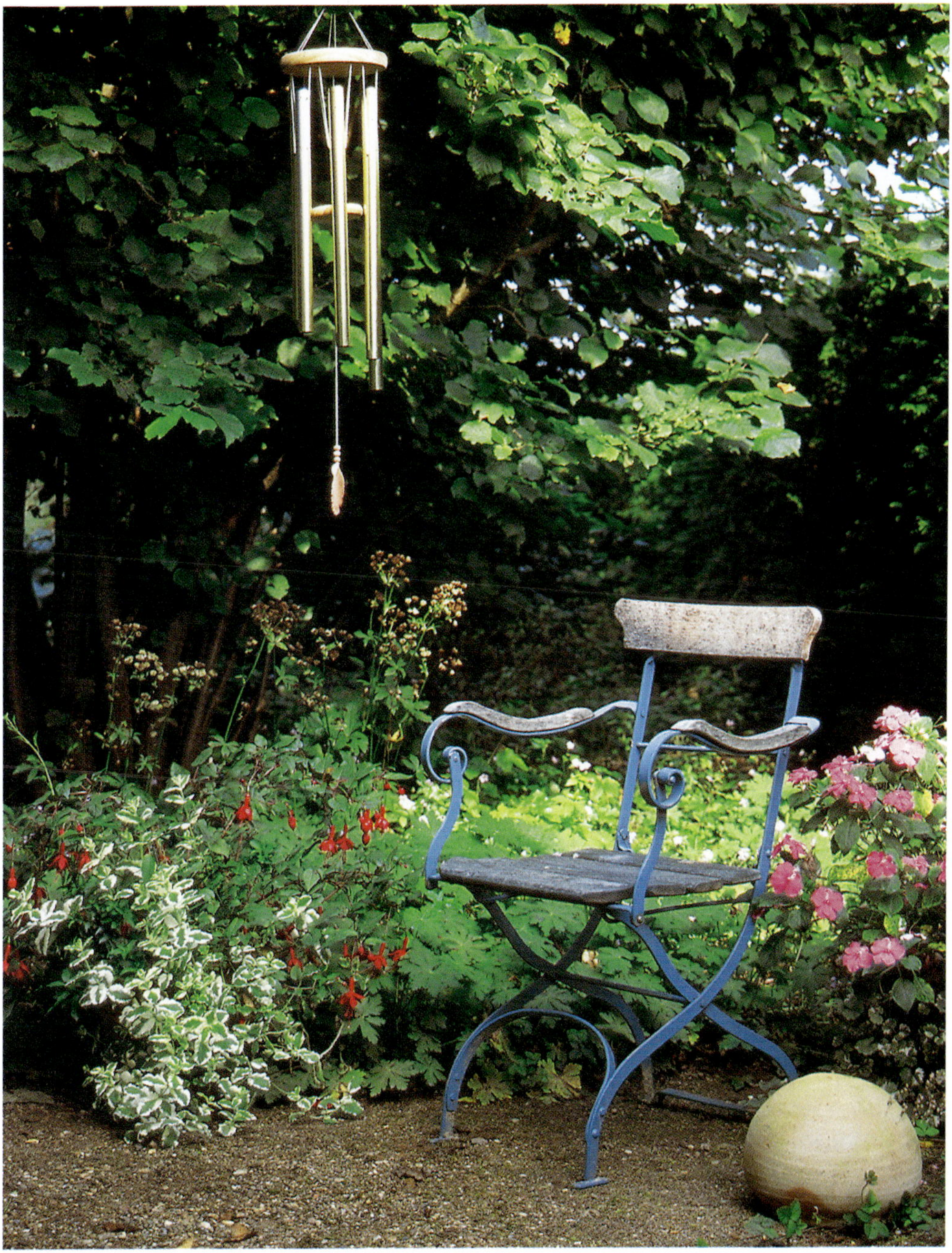

The Knowledge zone should be a calm retreat, somewhere to sit and contemplate.

Family

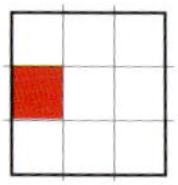

This zone lies to the left of the centre of the bagua. The element assigned to it (see p. 21) is Wood with the colours green and light to medium blue. The element Water has an encouraging effect along with the colours black to dark blue. The element Metal with the colours white, silver and gold has an inhibiting effect.
This zone says a lot about you and your relationships with your relatives, ancestors, superiors and authority figures. Do everything in your power to make sure this area is free of negative influences. Treat any diseased plants using organic methods, not harmful pesticides or fungicides and remove weeds and tree stumps as they represent unresolved problems and misdeeds. If you find it hard to take on new ideas or break free of your past, or if you feel your relations with parents, grandparents or siblings could be better, pay close attention to the balance in this zone.

Cosy sitting corners

This is one of the most favourable bagua zones for a seating area. Include comfortable seats for all the family – and make space here for family get-togethers in the garden. The only drawback is that as this zone is situated on the boundary of the property, it may not be very private and noise can penetrate from outside. If possible, construct a protective earth wall around the zone or frame it with a small group of mounds. If you plant hedges or bushes on the wall you will be sitting in a position that is relatively protected from observers, noise and wind.

Sunken sitting area

A sunken sitting area (see p. 4) will also provide protection. You will be able to descend via steps into a zone with a particularly pleasant, mild micro-climate that will also give you a feeling of shelter. Usually the side can be designed as a dry-stone wall in which many small creatures and insects will find shelter. As the element Earth is emphasised strongly with the sunken arrangement, and this element inhibits the zone's encouraging element Water, you should bring in Wood energy (see p. 22) through plants that will draw nutrients from the Earth. You could use wooden decking as an attractive and chi-enhancing alternative to the more conventional Earth-based patio materials. The horizontal slats of decking will act as a straight line to speed up the chi. A straight bench with wooden slats will have a similar energising effect, so try to keep a balance or you will never be able to relax in this zone. Use plenty of cushions to soften harsh lines, or choose rounded chairs with curved backs as they help the chi to flow smoothly and may prove far more relaxing.
A simple water feature will have an encouraging effect in this zone. Even a bird bath or a shallow trough will be beneficial.

Centre (Tai Chi)

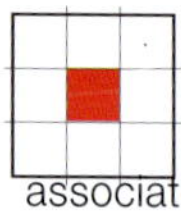

As the name indicates, this zone lies right in the centre of the bagua. The associated element is Earth with the colours yellow, orange and brown. The element Fire is supportive with the colours red, wine red and pink. Wood, with the colours green and light to medium blue, is inhibiting.
The position in the centre of your garden represents the life force and also the health of the inhabitants. The more open and energy-collecting you can make the design of this most important area, the more healing and centring vibrations will pour in from the surroundings.

The right design

In its simplest and most open form, the centre of the garden can be designed as a peaceful lawn area. Energy-collecting centres, however, are known from many classical knot and monastery gardens (see p. 8-9): they have a cross-path in the centre in which the different energy veins run together. The paths are often flanked by beds with a low-growing frame of plants that gently channel the energy. In the centre the focus is often provided by a circular bed with a striking arrangement of plants, a fountain or a sculpture with a particular radiative power, that will heighten the pulse of flowing energy. A spiral bed in the centre will demonstrate a similar effect. Do not bring too many objects and plants into the Centre that are associated with the element Wood as these draw too much energy from the earth and your Centre. If these kinds of objects are already present, you may be able to inhibit their effect (see p. 22).

No blockages

The Centre should be designed attractively but not be blocked with a massive constructed object. A little pavilion or summerhouse would, therefore, be better accommodated away from the centre of the garden. It would be ideal in the Partnership zone. On no account should a tool shed be situated in the Centre – it would be far better in the Knowledge zone (see p. 50).

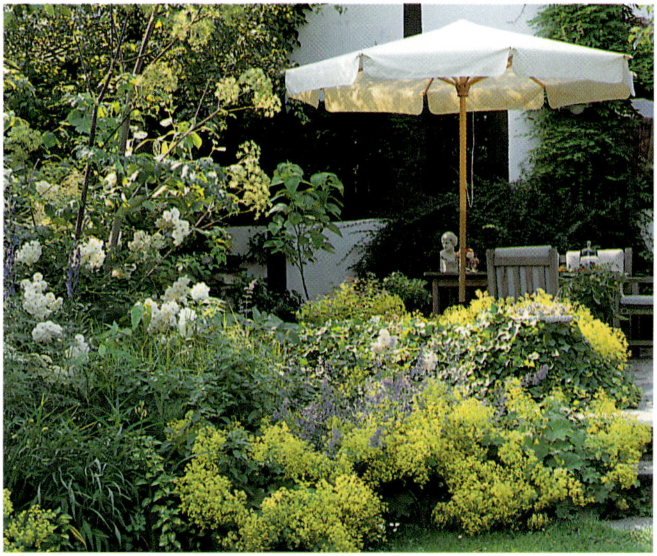

A spacious sitting area for the whole family.

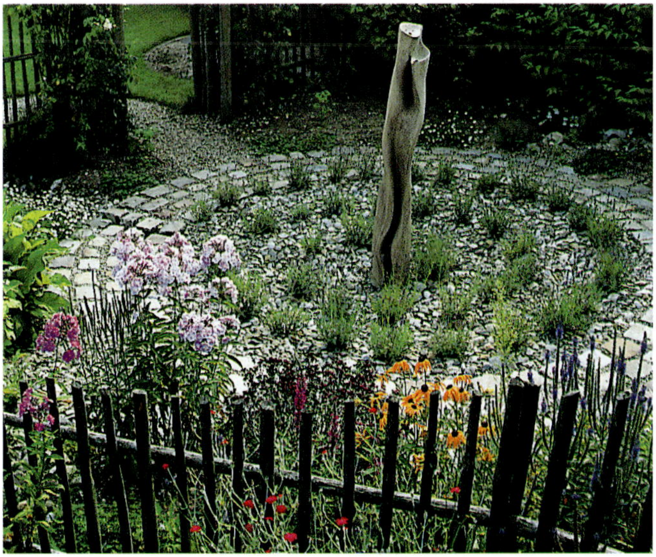

This circular bed and modern sculpture are ideal for the Centre zone.

Children

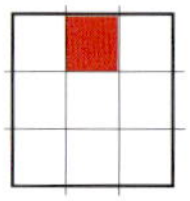

This zone lies right of the centre of the bagua. It is associated with the element Metal, the colours are white, silver and gold. The element Earth is supportive together with the colours yellow, orange and brown. The element Fire has an inhibiting effect with the colours pink, red and wine red.
This zone is the most active and creativity-enhancing in the whole garden, just as children bring much life into the family.

Children's playground

If you have children of your own, this is the best possible place for a children's play area that is as imaginative and full of fun as possible. The laughter and play of children and the joy with which they greet the new day allows cheerful energy to be created in their surroundings. You could also establish here a small, virtually undisturbed refuge for wildlife. These enchanted areas radiate a very special magic and small children in particular will be captivated by spending time in this part of the garden. Given the right conditions, the radiation from zones like these is strong enough to have a positive influence on the entire garden and even on the neighbouring gardens and buildings. You will find a much larger variety of species appearing in your garden and have noticeably fewer problems with pests.

Creativity and inspiration

If your children are grown up, or you have no children of your own you can still encourage creativity by placing unusual or inspiring works of art in this zone. Even a vegetable garden or a small scented garden will be favourable in this zone. Summer-scented plants like buddleia species will encourage butterflies and bees to come into your garden. The bees not only provide an important service by pollinating flowers, their orderly social structure will also harmonise the surroundings in which they spend time. In addition, many scented plants like tansy (*Phacelia tanacetifolia)* also deposit important nutrients in the soil.

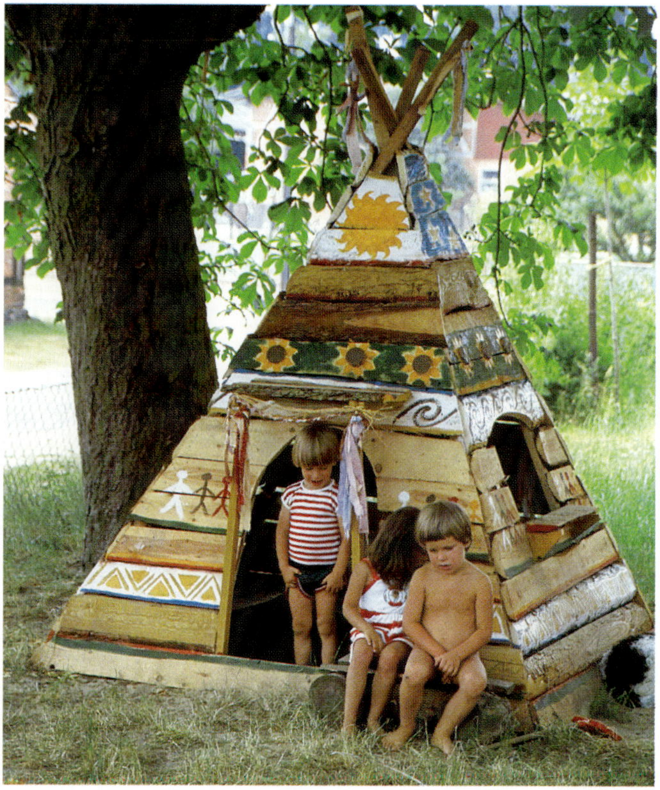

A cheerful play area for the children.

Wealth

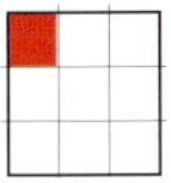

This zone lies in the left, back corner of the bagua. It is associated with the element Wood and the colours green and light blue to medium blue. Include plants such as clematis and juniper *(Juniperus communis)* here. The element Water is supportive together with the colours dark blue to black, while Metal is inhibiting with the colours white, silver and gold. This zone stands not only for financial wealth but also for the ideals of enriching events and experiences. This is a good place for tall accessories that strive upwards, like obelisks, columns or posts. As Water encourages wealth – and prosperity is associated with running water – a spring stone or a stream would be excellent in this position. The compost heap, which stands for future wealth, is least-suited to this garden position of all the possible ones.

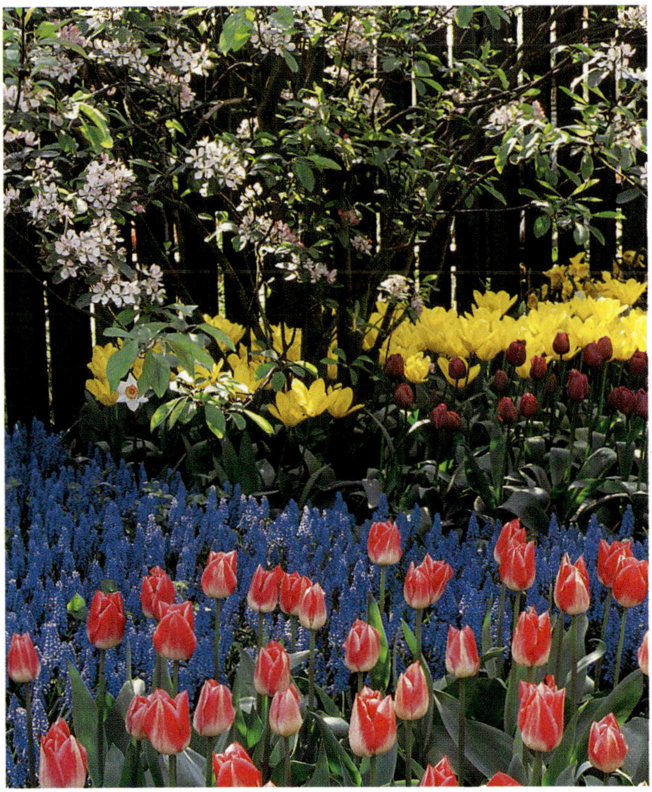

Splendid flowers for Wealth.

Fame

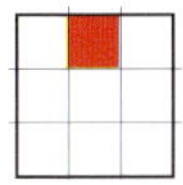

This zone lies at the centre back of the bagua. It is assigned to the element Fire and the colours pink, red and wine red. The element Wood is supportive together with the colours green and light to medium blue, and the element Water with the colours dark blue to black is inhibiting.
Your reputation and radiative power are reflected in this zone. Particularly beautiful, handsome plants or accessories like a sculpted figure are suitable for this area and will, in turn, nourish your personal charisma. A grill or barbecue would be good in this position. If you have a large area of water here make sure there is plenty of green in the surrounding area so that the Water nourishes the Wood and does not extinguish the flame of your Fame. Accessories like clay pots, paths made of gravel or flagstones that are associated with the element Earth will also inhibit the effect of Water.

Partnership

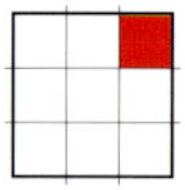

This zone lies back right in the bagua. It is associated with the element Earth and the colours yellow, orange and brown. The element Fire with the colours pink, red and wine red are supportive. The element Wood with the colours green and light to mid-blue are inhibiting. This particularly sensitive area supplies information on your relationships with your life partner, and also with friends, neighbours and colleagues. If plants suddenly begin to wither in this area of your garden, or are infested with pests, you should as quickly as possible pay a great deal of attention to your relationships. Very probably the condition of your plants will soon improve again.

Pergola and bower

Design this area with a pergola or a bower, as either of these will lend a special atmosphere to your garden and encourage communication and partnership aspects equally. Even a simple pergola with climbing plants, a construction made out of two vertical supports and a horizontal beam lying on top – like a gateway – will create a picturesque framework around a seat. If you require more of a visual screen, install further grids for plants to climb up and plant more climbers and creepers. To create shade around the sitting space, choose a bower with a number of wooden slats to create an airy but still protective, roof-like structure. For a particularly attractive arrangement, and if you have enough space, create a tunnel-like creeper-covered walkway with a hidden sitting area at the end of it. To build this, simply use several rose arches, regularly spaced one after the other.

Purchasing

Pergolas and bowers are best built of wood that can be obtained as a kit in a garden centre or builder's merchant's. They should not have too many sharp corners or points, as these will radiate cutting chi (see p. 10). If you are building it to last, do not drive the support beams straight into the ground as they would soon rot. There are various different kits you can get to anchor them and which enable you to screw the posts firmly into the soil at safe distances. These accessories should be obtainable at most good garden centres.

Greenery

Particularly beautiful, lasting species to cover pergolas and bowers with greenery in this zone can be found among climbing roses (*Rosa* species), honeysuckle (*Lonicera caprifolium*) or the yellow brown flowering *Aristolochia macrophylla* with its very large, heart-shaped leaves that provide a good visual screen. Among the annuals, the particularly fast-growing *Thunbergia alata* and *Ipomoea purpurea* are very suitable. Place plants in the surrounding area too, using low-growing species so that the structure does not look so isolated in the garden and provides a comfortable, secure feeling.

Pavilions

A pavilion is ideal for the partnership zone as it encourages harmonious relationships. By contrast with a summerhouse, a pavilion has a more open structure and will offer views to all sides through windows or openings. When you are sitting in it, you will still be protected from the weather and also from curious glances, provided there is enough plant cover. Pavilions can be obtained in self-assembly kits from good garden centres.

Light

As 'fiery' accessories encourage the Partnership zone, you should also place lamps in this area. If there is no mains connection nearby, you can use solar-powered lamps that are charged up during the daytime and are then switched on with a sensory switch at dusk and will last for a few hours.

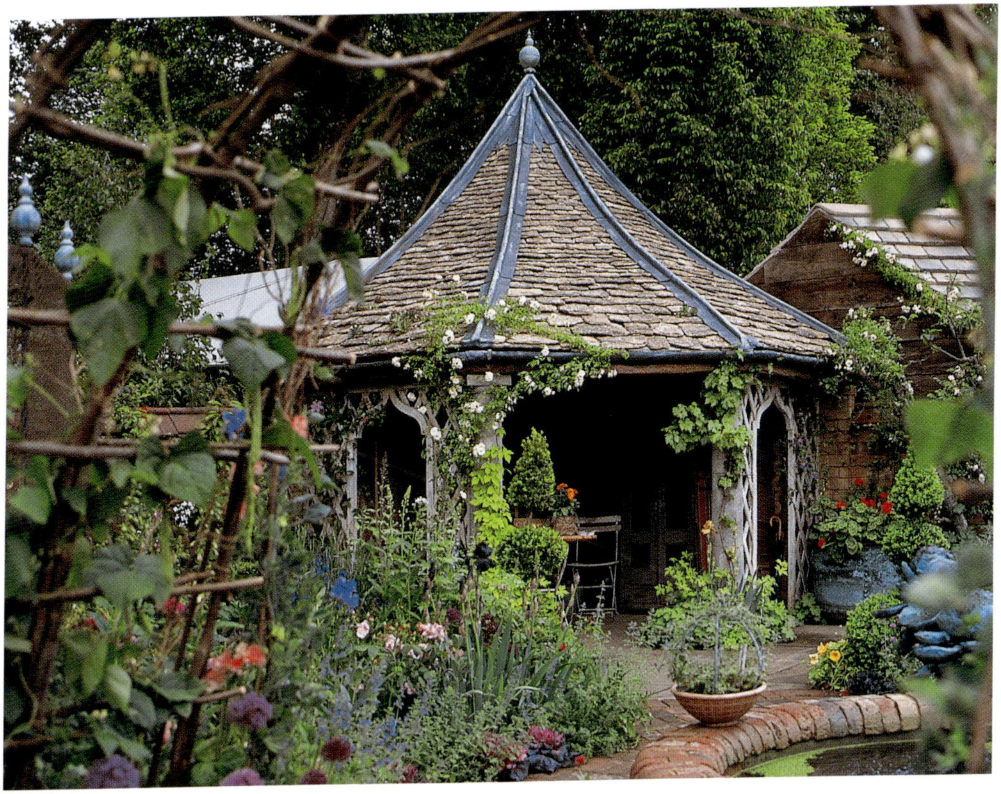

A pavilion for harmonious relationships.

In this zone, reduce or avoid (see p. 22) free-standing lampposts, flag poles or column-shaped plants that are associated with the element Wood and would draw energy away from the Earth.

Pairing

The Partnership zone can be beautifully accentuated with plants or accessories arranged in pairs. Place plants or use globes and garden lamps symmetrically positioned at each side of a path or seat. Think of the man/woman symbology and, if possible, avoid the impression of hierarchy or imbalance.

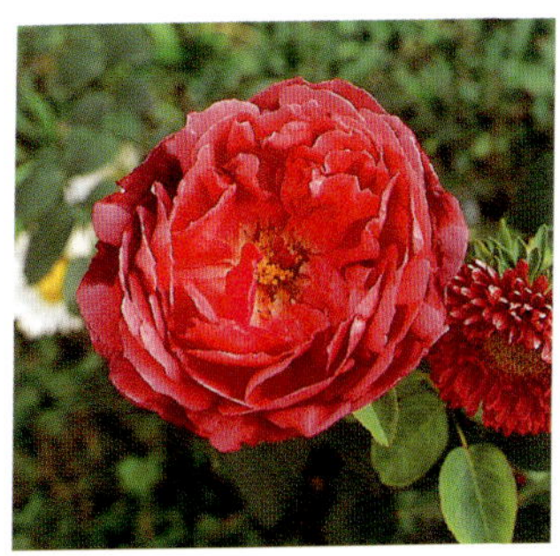

Roses for love.

Index

Subject and plant index

Numbers in **bold** indicate colour photographs and illustrations.

Index

Index

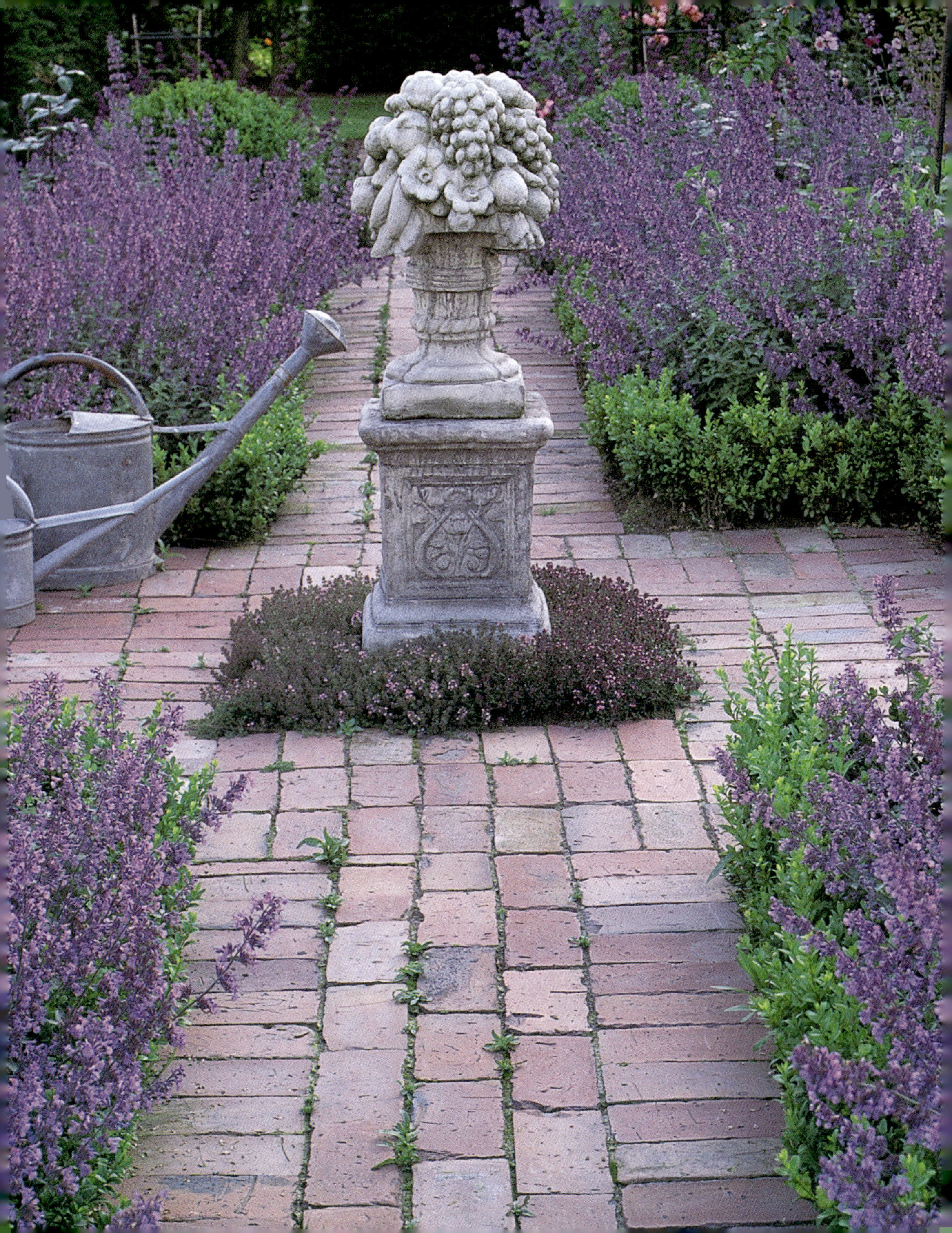

Further reading, credits, addresses

Further reading

If the books are unobtainable in bookshops, try libraries.
Guinness, Bunny, *Family Gardens*, ISBN 0-7153-0422-4, David & Charles, Newton Abbot
Jay, Roni, *Feng Shui In Your Garden*, ISBN 0-7225-3621-6, Thorsons, London
Rossbach, Sarah and Master Lin Yun, *Feng Shui Design*, ISBN 0-283-06324-6, Sidgwick & Jackson, London
Recht, Christine, *Success With Herbs,* ISBN 1-85391-396-0, Merehurst, London
Hale, Gill, *The Feng Shui Garden*, ISBN 185-410-5469, Aurum Press, London
Waring, Philippa, *The Feng Shui of Gardening,* ISBN 0-28-5634-364, Souvenir Press, London
Don, Monty, *The Sensuous Garden*, ISBN 1-85029-862-9, Conran Octopus, London
Brookes, John, *The New Garden,* ISBN 0-7513-0367-4, Dorling Kindersley, London

Acknowledgements

The author and the publishers wish to thank landscape architects Marion and Anton Robl in Daberg 9, 93437 Furth Im Wald, for their valuable comments. They designed the gardens illustrated on p. 4, 35 and 53 bottom.

Photographic acknowledgements

Atelier Dreiseitl: p. 32 bottom right, back cover; Becker: p. 2, 9 bottom, 33 bottom right, 49 centre right, 61; Borstell: front cover, bottom right, inside front cover, 9 top, 14/15, 20, 28/29, 29 right, 31, 32 top right, centre right, bottom left, 33 top, bottom left, 37 centre left, 43 top, 46/47, 55; Englbrecht: p. 41, 49 bottom, 57 bottom; Hofmeister: p. 4/5, 35 top, bottom, 53 bottom;
mein schöner Garten: Kögel/p. 49 top left;
mein schöner Garten: Krieg/ p. 49 top right;
Murdoch books: front cover, centre right;
Nickig: front cover, main picture, p. 3 right, 15 right, 37 centre centre, centre right, 39, 53 top;
Redeleit: front cover, top right, p. 5 right, 7, 37 top left, 40 left, right, 43 bottom, 49 centre left, 51, 54, inside back cover; Reinhard: p. 45 top,bottom; Strauss: p. 3 left, 47 right, 57 top;
Tschakert: p. 32 top left, 37 top right.

Suppliers

Gazing balls or mirror balls, as they are sometimes known, can be obtained from the following companies:
Esoterica, 5A Devonshire Road, Chiswick, London W4 2EU. Telephone 0181 994 1414.
Farbglashutte Lauscha GmbH, Strasse des Friedens 39, D-98724 Lauscha, Germany. Telephone 036702-281-0.
Glasblaserie Dieter Kunze, Haupstr. 35, D-78595, Hausen ob Verena. Telephone 07424-501793.

Warning and notes

This volume deals with the planning and designing of a feng shui garden. It provides inspiration and ideas on how you can make simple alterations in your garden to create an area of regeneration, peace and energy and influence your life positively. Feng shui encourages general well-being but is not a method for treating physical or emotional problems. In such cases expert advice should be sought. Some of the plants recommended here are toxic to varying degrees and they are identified as such in the tables on p. 21 and in the text. Make absolutely sure that children and domestic pets do not eat these plants or parts of them.
If you should sustain injuries while working in the garden with soil, please consult a doctor to discuss whether a vaccination against tetanus might be necessary.

Cover photographs

Front cover: (main picture) The *perfect way to enjoy a feng shui garden, in a hammock with the scents, sounds and sights of nature all around you.*
Front cover inset pictures: (top) Attractive garden accessories have a strengthening effect on many areas; (centre) annual sweet peas for scent and colour; (bottom) by simply walking under a rose arch you restore your energy levels.
Inside front cover: A true garden of the senses should contain splendid scented flowers and tasty fruit.
Back cover: A sitting place where you can recharge lost energy.

Reprinted 2000
This edition published in 1999 by
Merehurst Limited
Ferry House
51-57 Lacy Road,
Putney, London,
SW15 1PR

ISBN 1-85391-792-3

A catalogue record for this book is available from the British Library.

Translated by
Astrid Mick
Edited by
Karen Douthwaite
Typeset by
Anita Ruddell
Printed in Hong Kong by Wing King Tong

A place for relaxing in peace

The Far-Eastern teaching of feng shui creates no boundaries to the imagination when it comes to designing a space that is protected from noise and curious glances. Such a place is particularly favoured in the bagua zone of Knowledge. In its most simple form, a space can be created by just setting up a comfortable chair in a spot that is surrounded by pleasant plants. But a special cave-like sitting place, surrounded by woody plants is ideal and is just the place to switch off and recover from everyday stress.

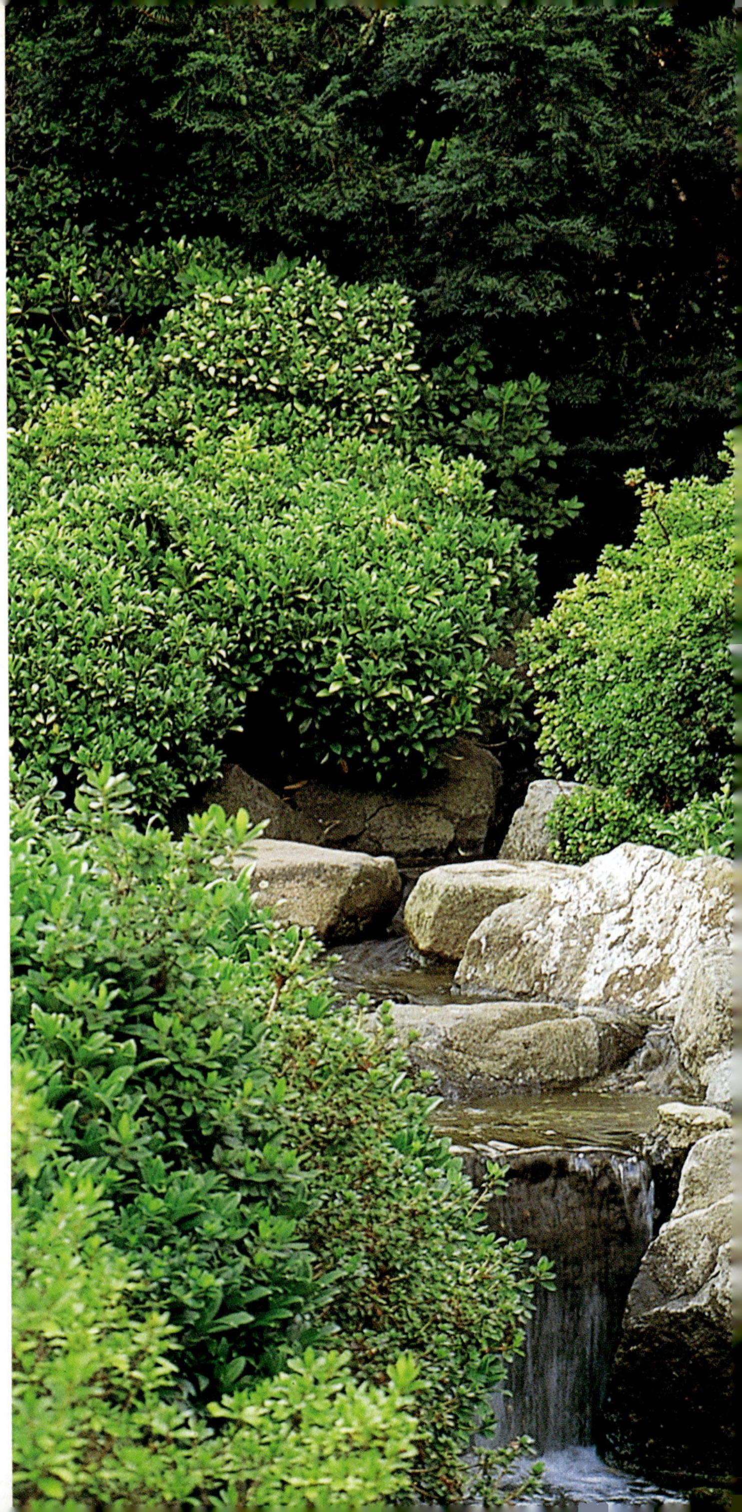

A simple cushion placed on a rounded boulder beside a stream invites you to sit and think. The gentle splashing of the stream and the harmonious sounds of the wind chimes provide an intense atmosphere for contemplation.